MW01069369

FOOD *for* MENOPAUSE

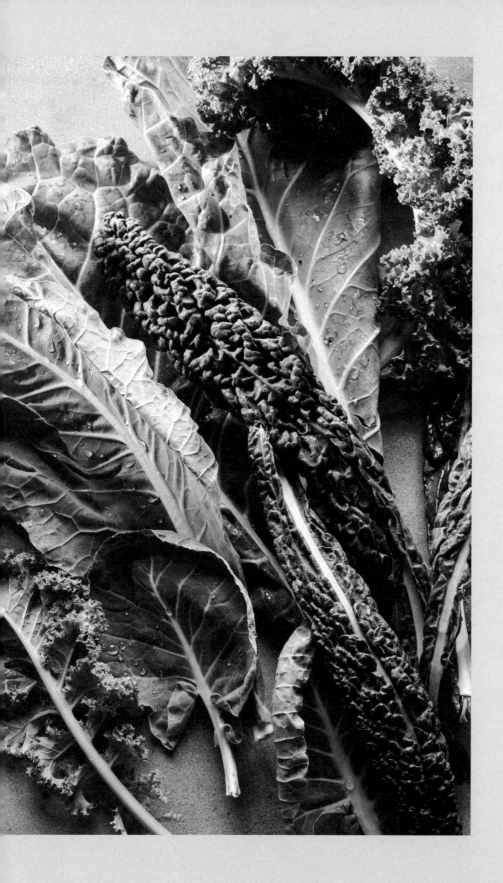

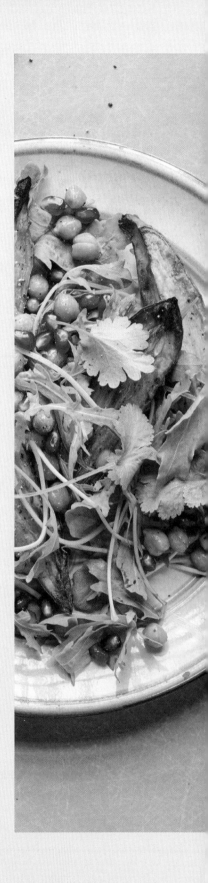

Dr Linia Patel PhD, RD

FOOD *for* MENOPAUSE

Recipes and nutritional advice
for perimenopause, menopause
and beyond

murdoch books
London | Sydney

To my beloved mama ... and all the women like her who endured the menopause phase of life without the right tools and support.

Contents

Introduction

I'm sitting in my London clinic and my client, Olivia, is in front of me. She is 44, a mum of three and the global managing director at a top consultancy firm. She tells me that she has gone from juggling a high-flying job in the city, travelling the world and co-parenting three children to having waves of panic before every meeting as she has started to completely blank out at points she is expected to deliver. It's like a chunk of her brain has shut down, she explains, and it's beginning to rock her sense of identity. She's trying her best to power through but she has reached a breaking point. It's as though she, the go-getter who used to thrive under pressure, has been ambushed overnight by a sudden inability to deal with anything – even the simple tasks.

Jess's story is the same but different. She is 45 years old and lives with her boyfriend. Over the past year, Jess told me that, despite her healthy-ish approach to nutrition and exercise, she had started noticing subtle changes to her body and mood. At first, she attributed this to general life events. She had just bought a new house with her boyfriend, and she was playing with the idea of going freelance. She came to see me because the exercise and nutrition routines that had worked to get her into shape in the past just didn't seem to cut it anymore. It seemed that even if she tried to watch what she was eating, she put on weight. Her bloated belly now felt out of control. She didn't want to have sex and this was becoming an issue in her relationship.

As a women's health dietitian, I work with women on a daily basis and I have the privilege of hearing hundreds of stories. Too many women in their forties are struggling with their health and life feels hard.

SCAN THIS QR CODE TO UNLOCK
ONLINE CONTENT, VIDEOS AND MORE

LINIAPATELNUTRITION

'The night sweats mean I'm changing my sheets daily.'

'Something is not right.'

'Sex is so painful.'

'I am constantly in raging bitch mode. I feel so angry all the time. I hate who I am becoming.'

'I've lost myself.'

'I'm experiencing a soul-crushing sadness.'

'I feel flat. I'm self-medicating with sugar.'

'I'm losing my hair. It has become so thin. I'm getting worried something is seriously wrong.'

'I have been told I have prediabetes. It's a wake-up call.'

'I feel as though a tyre has been sewn into my waist.'

If any of this resonates with you, then know it's okay and that you are not alone. While all these stories are unique, to some extent they are the same. There is a common theme. All these women are experiencing the profound effect of a midlife hormone flux. Add to that the fact that we are the 'do-it-all' generation: the conscious mother, a kind carer to aging parents, a fun friend, the career women, a beauty queen, a self-care guru and a user of environmentally friendly menstrual cups. Societal demands also push us to pretend we all have the perfect Instagrammable life. It can get pretty intense, right?

While you may have once been able to seamlessly manage the juggle and the pressure of adulting, add in the midlife hormone factor and the impact is waaay bigger. You feel it more.

Menopause affects 100 per cent of women assigned female at birth. More than half of the world's population will experience it. Yet most women say they are not prepared. And another 75 per cent report not knowing that what they eat and how they live has an impact on their symptoms. Until recently, many of these symptoms were written off as part of a natural part of aging, something that women simply had to tough out and live with. And being women … we just did and carried on!

However, there is no need for Olivia, Jess or anyone to suffer unnecessarily with symptoms – or to reach a breaking point before getting help. Growing up and aging are inevitable.

Gaining weight, being utterly overwhelmed, crippled with anxiety, not sleeping and having a below-zero libido isn't.

We now understand more about what happens to women's hormones as we age and how best to adapt to the changes and, ultimately, to thrive.

Yes, midlife is full on. Yes, your body is changing. That is the reality. But therein lies the opportunity. There is an upside. Getting older has its perks, too. Surveys asking women about the benefits of aging report that most women find that, with age, it is easier to speak their mind, they worry less about other people's opinions and, overall, they have clearer priorities. Imagine if we harnessed the increased emotional and social intelligence (what we call wisdom) and gained health intelligence too? The menopause years are an opportunity to do just that. To get to know yourself. Know yourself so that you can manage your symptoms. Know yourself so that you can be an active participant in determining how you age. Know yourself so that you can stretch and not snap. Know yourself so that you can show up as the best version of you.

Now this is something my forty-something self thinks is quite awesome.

In general, women's health is often under-explored and under-researched, but the narrative is changing. There is now more information on the menopause than ever before, which is brilliant. However,

I want to empower you ... so you can manage your symptoms, feel like yourself again and get the most out of your body.

even with this increasing level of available information, women's lifestyle is missing from the conversation. Women in my clinic and on various social media platforms are hungry (pun intended) for practical advice on what they should be putting on their plates.

With this book I wanted to create a toolkit for women in their forties and beyond to help you understand what is going on but, more importantly, to give you practical and effective strategies to make the journey easier. Being both a Women's Health Dietitian and a Performance Nutritionist (and maybe having sprinkles of overachieving tendencies myself), I also want to empower you to take it up a level, so you can manage your symptoms, feel like yourself again and get the most out of your body.

The term 'performance' can seem hard core and slightly scary, right? It shouldn't. On the simplest level, performance nutrition is all about improving your biology so you can get more out of your life. It's about unlocking your power. Optimising your potential. Being the best version of you.

Hormones are the things in our bodies that make us tick. They run and regulate our bodies, acting as chemical messengers. They help get stuff done. So, if you learn to eat to make your hormones work for you rather than against you, you are onto something.

Now this isn't about making you into superwoman. If you are all about kicking ass, great. This book is for you!

If you are already experiencing perimenopausal/menopausal symptoms and simply want to manage them and feel more like yourself again, this book is for you too. If you are already menopausal and want to know how to eat for the second half of life, this book is also for you. If you are just approaching your forties, this book is for you too. Menopause nutrition is probably not top of your list of things to figure out this week. It's easy to think of menopause as distant, something you worry about down the line, but you may be surprised at how high priority – even for the spring chickens among us – it is. Studies show that the way you prepare yourself during your late thirties and early forties is the game changer.

And, in the spirit of being inclusive: gents, this book is for you too. We all need to be aware. Women and men, young, old and anything in-between, because we all have a woman in our lives (mother, sister, partner, friend, colleague) and having everyone recognise and understand the menopause is so important in helping to change the narrative around it.

How to use this book

Every woman goes through the menopause, but her experience is unique to her. While tailored nutritional advice is the gold standard, there are fundamental science-based frameworks that can guide you. These will allow you to understand yourself better and empower you to tailor your approach to your own personal symptoms, experience and circumstances.

I want to make this book as practical as possible. I'm a busy woman, too – juggling life, work and a relationship. I don't always have time during the week to spend hours preparing gourmet food – let's be real. But I do eat well and I love good food. That's exactly what this book and my recipes are about – being realistic, yet learning to nourish and feed your body to maximise your hormones and your health. There are four parts to this book.

Part 1: Understanding your body and your symptoms

Understanding what's changing, why it's happening and how to deal with it can make the whole process a lot less frustrating and uncomfortable. Here, we get to know some key hormones, understand what they do, how they change over time and how this affects your body and the way you feel.

Part 2: Eating for success

Here you'll learn the key nutrition pillars, what the top foods are to include in your diet and what your plate needs to look like most of the time.

Part 3: Living for success

You can eat the best diet in the world, but if you don't get on top of these other core pillars then you won't be #winning. I've given you a toolbox of practical ideas that you can use to help you deal with your symptoms and support your menopause journey.

Part 4: Recipes for success

I have 81 delicious recipes to choose from to take you through breakfast, lunch, dinner and the weekend, along with lots of tips and ways to change them up to suit your goals, your family circumstances and whether or not you eat meat.

I am a highlighter and underliner and I would suggest that you do this for the chapters and topics that feel most relevant to you, so you can come back to them. I have also created a bit of a pick-and-mix approach as you will find that your journey morphs and changes along the way and, over time, other sections may become more relevant to you. I can't wait for you to read it, and to see you using the tips and trying the recipes too.

You've got this!

Big love.

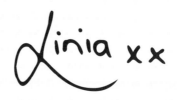

PART 1

Understanding your body and your symptoms

Your hormone masterclass

There are around 200 different hormones in the human body. They act like chemical messengers that help to get stuff done. They help regulate various organs and systems. They regulate things like your heart rate, your mood, when you sleep, when you wake up, your appetite, your digestion, your sex drive, how excited or relaxed or motivated you feel, and, of course, things like your menstrual cycle and your ability to have a baby. Each hormone in the body has an optimal level to maintain hormone balance. All these delicately controlled levels of hormones then all work together, like a finely tuned orchestra.

From your forties onwards there are groups of hormones that it's important you know about as they have a big impact on your overall health. Learning about these hormones will help you understand some of the changes that happen in your body and will also empower you to know which ones you need to work to keep in check or boost, so that you can not only ease your symptoms but also age well. I want to introduce you to your most important hormones when it comes to menopause:

> **Female hormones:** Progesterone, oestrogen and testosterone
> **Stress hormones:** Cortisol and adrenaline
> **'Happy' hormones:** Dopamine and serotonin.

Of course, there are other important hormones that I want you to know the names of, as I will be talking about these as well. These other hormones include oxytocin, endorphins, melatonin, dehydroepiandrosterone (DHEA), thyroid hormones and insulin.

Female hormones

Progesterone, oestrogen and testosterone are called steroid hormones and are some of the most active hormones in your body. Progesterone and oestrogen are produced mainly in the ovaries and, in smaller amounts, from the adrenal glands and the placenta (if you are pregnant) and they work as a team. Progesterone and oestrogen levels rise and fall at different points in a woman's menstrual cycle and at different points in a woman's life. When they are at the correct levels they act like a seesaw and balance each other out.

Sex hormones do what they say on the tin – they support our reproductive needs. However, their roles are not just linked to baby-making and it is this whole spectrum of other roles that you should be aware of.

PROGESTERONE

Let's unpack progesterone first. Progesterone is the pro-pregnancy hormone. It prepares the body for pregnancy and supports the developing embryo. However, did you know that it also has a profound influence on our brain and mood?

Dubbed the 'relaxing' hormone, progesterone helps to calm the brain and boost your mood. It stimulates your brain to produce a neurotransmitter (a chemical that has an effect on your brain) called

Oestrogen is your extrovert, a seeker of attention and sassy socialite that loves a good party.

gamma-aminobutyric acid (GABA). The higher your level of progesterone, the more GABA you produce. Goodbye anxiety and mood swings, hello to a calm mind. Progesterone also helps you remember things and be more on the ball in terms of learning and it helps regulate sleep.

Many health professionals use analogies to make hormone-talk more relatable. Some refer to different hormones as key instruments within an orchestra. Giving our hormones characters is a concept that resonates with me personally. If progesterone had a character, she would be a bit of an introvert, a little shy, yet wonderfully calm, cool and collected.

OESTROGEN

Oestrogen is the second female hormone that is integral to womanhood. There are three types of oestrogen circulating in our bloodstream: estrone (E1), oestradiol (E2) and estriol (E3). Although they all play a major role in the development and function of the female reproductive system, each one has slightly different functions. For ease, I will refer to oestrogen collectively. In reproductive terms, oestrogen drives the 'building' of tissues, such as the womb lining, in preparation for pregnancy. One thing is for sure: it's a hormone that needs a better PR team as oestrogen has some wide-ranging, far-reaching functions that a lot of us don't know about.

When you scan the body for oestrogen receptors, you will find them not only in the reproductive tract and the breasts, but also in tissues like bones, the brain, liver, intestine, skin, urinary tract, blood vessels and salivary glands (I know, it's crazy, right?!). Where there is a receptor, there is a role. So this means that, in the right balance, oestrogen can do the following:

1. **It impacts your appetite.** It makes you feel hungrier. This is why on the days leading up to your period, when oestrogen levels in your body are super high, you may feel hungrier than normal and have some cravings.

2. **It keeps your skin supple.** Think of that pregnancy glow, when oestrogen levels are at their peak! However, too much can cause acne.

3. **It affects your mind in all manner of ways.** So much so that researchers still don't fully understand the implication of oestrogen on our mood. What we do know is that the drop in oestrogen may be one of the reasons that women experience postpartum depression as levels of oestrogen plummet dramatically from their elevated state during pregnancy.

4. **It bolsters your bones.** Along with vitamin D and calcium, oestrogen forms part of the dream team that helps you to maintain strong bones for life. It helps the body to repair and rebuild bone.

5. **It helps you sleep.** Oestrogen plays a role in the metabolism of serotonin and other neurotransmitters that affect our sleep-wake cycle.

6. **It keeps your vagina moist.** It also increases your sex drive.

7. **It keeps your heart healthy.** It keeps cholesterol in check and your blood vessels nice and elastic.

8. **It determines where fat is stored.** Hips, thighs and breasts are oestrogen's preference.

9. It's involved in blood-sugar control. It supports insulin (more on this important hormone later) to usher blood sugars into the cells.

10. It's neuroprotective. This is an area I am personally invested in as I watched my beloved mum struggle with dementia. It was very tough. Some research suggests oestrogen in the brain is thought to support the grey matter, the part of our central nervous system that allows us to control movement, memory and emotions, and the part that is heavily affected in conditions like Alzheimer's and dementia. But oestrogen doesn't just help with behaviour, it also has a general nourishing and protective role. There is so much more we need to learn to fully understand the whole picture here.

I could go on. But I think you get the idea of how integral oestrogen is and why we may experience so many symptoms as we age and have lower levels of this hormone.

Character-wise, oestrogen is your extrovert, a seeker of attention and sassy socialite that loves a good party. In the right dose she is loved by everyone but she can get a bit too much and be a real troublemaker (keep that point in your mind) and that is why she needs progesterone as a BFF to keep her in check and bring out the best in her.

TESTOSTERONE

You may think of testosterone as a hormone that only men produce, but women produce it too. We only have about one-tenth of the testosterone levels that men have but its effects are still powerful. In a woman, testosterone is produced by the ovaries and adrenal glands. It affects many different things, from your mood, your energy levels and your brain's ability to focus through to your muscle strength and tone. Testosterone has an important role in your sex life, too. It affects your clitoris's size, your sex drive and orgasms.

Stress hormones

There are two glands that sit on top of your kidneys called the adrenal glands. Your adrenal glands are like protective bodyguards. They are there to keep you safe. If they sense danger, they release a cascade of stress hormones, adrenaline (also called noradrenaline) and cortisol being the most important. Imagine the nervous energy you get just before a presentation or something that takes you out of your comfort zone, where you experience your heart pounding and maybe even break a little bit of a sweat. That's adrenaline for you. It gives you a rush of energy so that you can run as fast as you can and get the hell out of the situation or brace yourself and fight back, should you need to. If adrenalineis released in short bursts, it can be helpful. It switches on 'performance' mode.

You don't feel the effects of cortisol straight away. Our bodies actually release cortisol once every 24 hours in a pulse around 30 minutes after we wake up – to help get you out of bed and get going. So, while cortisol is often thought of as the 'bad' guy, it's important to remember that your body needs some cortisol. In the correct amount, it's a great motivating hormone that keeps you nice and alert. Chronic stress, which results in excessive amounts of cortisol being released, is what puts pressure on our adrenal glands. It causes a different reaction in our body. Think of cortisol as a friend you couldn't live without but who is best enjoyed in small doses. In general, a little stress helps us perform well, but chronic stress is exhausting and takes a toll on our body.

'Happy' hormones

As humans, we all strive to be happy. While there are different definitions of happiness, in the simplest definition, happiness is about having positive emotions and being content. The reason we feel upbeat, chirpy or elated is due to complex chemical reactions that happen within your body involving (you guessed it) hormones. I am no neuroscientist and I want to make things relatable for you, so keep in mind I am giving you a simplified explanation. Of course, there is a complicated nature to happiness and things can't be isolated to single hormones. It's about their overall interaction.

The hormones that give you the happiness factor (H factor) include:

> **dopamine**
> **serotonin**
> **oxytocin**
> **endorphins.**

Dopamine is called your 'feel-good hormone'. Praised on a job? Hello, dopamine. Reward and pleasure are the most established roles of dopamine. Dopamine motivates you to want to have a good experience again. Unexpected rewards have a greater dopamine release. Dopamine also helps you to focus and allows you to learn new things and remember them. It can be released when you do things such as listening to your favourite tune, getting a massage and exercising – or gambling, taking drugs or online shopping. Since too much dopamine can encourage addictive behaviour, it's a balancing act.

Serotonin is our mood stabiliser. It makes us feel cosy, safe and content. It helps to regulate your sleep and wake cycle and is linked to how well your brain learns and how regular your bowel movement is. The amazing thing about serotonin is that 95 per cent of your body's levels are produced in your intestine by your gut bacteria. Serotonin is naturally triggered by things we do each day, like being in the sunshine (particularly in the morning), getting a good night's sleep, spending time in nature and other self-care activities that refill your tank.

Often called the 'love' or 'cuddle' hormone, oxytocin is all about bonding and forming attachments. So it is an essential part of childbirth, creating a strong parent–child bond and increasing closeness and positive relationship feelings in general. Simply being attracted to someone can lead to the production of oxytocin. But cuddles, kisses, sex and orgasms also contribute to oxytocin production. Women are thought to be more affected by oxytocin than men.

And the exercise 'high' is real. Endorphins are neurotransmitters released by the body that act as your body's natural painkillers. They give your body a sense of euphoria which reduces stress and covers any pain. They are released in response to pain or stress but also during activities like exercise.

YOUR HORMONES ARE ALL LINKED

In the hormone world, everything links together. Like an orchestra, a sophisticated communication system made up of the hypothalamic-pituitary-adrenal axis (HPA axis) works hard to keep all your systems in balance. The HPA axis is the system through which the brain and adrenal glands communicate. This master regulator takes into consideration several different factors and cues from internal signals and the world around us, which then influences how much and which of these hormones are released. This then influences, and in turn is influenced by, your age, what and how much you eat, your activity and your stress levels.

How your hormones change with age

The first thing to highlight is that what we think happens as we age and the reality is often a tad different. There are some distinct stages that the female hormones go through, which generally work as a linear process. However, there is always the individual dimension.

Understanding the different hormonal stages women go through will help you know what to expect on your journey, how to manage your symptoms as they arrive and, importantly, know when it's time to talk to your GP or a healthcare professional. Your power lies in being proactive.

According to the American Society for Reproductive Medicine's Stages of Reproductive Aging, a woman's life can be delineated into distinct stages, from the onset of menstrual cycles through the reproductive age to the menopause and post menopause.

Let's start from the very beginning. When we are born as females, we have about two million eggs in our ovaries.

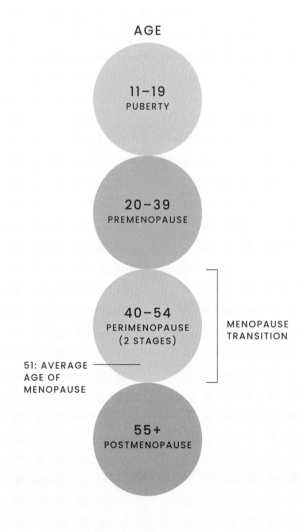

AGE

11–19
PUBERTY

20–39
PREMENOPAUSE

40–54
PERIMENOPAUSE
(2 STAGES)

MENOPAUSE
TRANSITION

51: AVERAGE
AGE OF
MENOPAUSE

55+
POSTMENOPAUSE

We can transform this natural transition into a milestone that is not feared but celebrated.

By puberty, through a natural process of controlled cell death (called apoptosis), this number reduces to about 300,000–500,000 eggs. Somewhere in our teenage years, our ovaries kick in and begin to produce the main female hormones, oestrogen and progesterone. This cues the development of boobs, hips ... and the menstrual cycle. Technically, the start of your periods is called menarche. Under normal conditions, an egg is released during each menstrual cycle and, if it doesn't get fertilised by a strong-swimming sperm, we have a monthly period.

During this cycle, oestrogen and progesterone go from low levels (luteal phase) to elevated levels (follicular phase) before dropping again. This drop is what causes a woman's menstrual cycle. The rise and fall of both hormones is also why you feel different from week to week and day to day throughout the cycle.

From your early twenties, oestrogen hits its prime as your body enters its reproductive years. From your thirties, you start to experience a slow and gradual decrease in your hormones. Testosterone, for example, starts to decline 1–2 per cent per year from your thirties. This can lead to a gradual loss of muscle mass and will mean you put on weight more easily if you are not proactive.

From about 35 to forty, you are in the premenopausal stage. Although it's not an officially recognised medical term or an official stage of the menopause, shifts in our hormones begin in this phase and the biological clock ticks more loudly. The egg count in the female body continues to decrease. As ovarian reserves decrease, so do a female's hormones.

Oestrogen is the hormone responsible for fertility decreases, but it's actually progesterone that takes a bigger toll first. In this phase you will still have periods – whether they are regular or irregular – and you are still in your reproductive years. Although there are hormonal changes, for the most part there are no noticeable changes in your body.

From your forties, you begin to approach the menopause. Society's influence on menopause may have conjured up images of old maids for us all. It used to be seen as something scary, so scary that our grandmothers and mothers didn't talk about it much. It was referred to as 'the change', an inevitable, painful fate that women resigned themselves to endure.

No, girl! It's time to change the narrative. Big time. And in order to do this we need to understand what happens, take note and then be empowered with key hacks to support and balance our unique female physiology so that we can transform this natural transition into a milestone that is not feared but celebrated.

A growing number of famous women are getting real about menopause and speaking openly about their journeys. And thankfully the narrative around it is changing – albeit slowly. The reality is that women in the midlife are more powerful than ever. You can be in your midlife and still be smashing it. Thanks, J.Lo, Halle Berry, Michelle Obama!

What exactly is the menopause?

'Menopause' is very often used as an umbrella term to encompass all the changes a woman goes through as her body prepares to, and finally stops, menstruating. But menopause is not a single event; it is the second of three stages a woman experiences in her menopause years. The menopause transition broadly involves three phases.

1. Perimenopause. 'Peri' in Greek means 'around' – so perimenopause means around the menopause. It is the phase leading up to the menopause when our hormone system is in a state of flux. So this is the phase where we begin to experience some of the symptoms of the menopause. However, if you are not aware of it, the symptoms can easily be written off as a result of 'life' and make you struggle unnecessarily. These hormonal changes start to happen much earlier than many women realise and can last from four years to a decade. What makes this phase so difficult to detect is that there is no specific age when the symptoms start to occur. Most females begin to experience symptoms in their mid to late forties.

2. Menopause. Officially, the menopause is the point at which you have not had a period for twelve consecutive months. On average, in the UK and USA it is at 51 years. However, the exact age varies for each woman. It's kind of like the delivery person who says they'll be there between 9am and 8pm — it's a bit hard to predict and can be influenced by several factors (more on that later).

3. Postmenopause. Technically this begins when you have not had a period for twelve months and one day. This stage signals the end of your reproductive years. While your ovaries produce low levels of oestrogen and progesterone, you will no longer ovulate or menstruate.

STAGES IN A WOMAN'S REPRODUCTIVE LIFE
- *Menarche: The point when you begin your menstrual cycle.*
- *Premenopause: When hormones are slowly declining, before menopausal symptoms start.*
- *Perimenopause: When you still have your period and begin to experience some menopausal symptoms. It can be split into early and late perimenopause.*
- *Menopause: When you have not had a period for twelve consecutive months.*
- *Postmenopause: The rest your life after your menopause.*
- *Premature menopause: For most females, the menopause begins from the age of forty. However, it can start earlier for individuals who experience premature ovarian failure or who have surgical removal of both ovaries at a young age.*

When will I start the menopause?

The menopause journey can last anywhere from two to fourteen years but typically lasts around four to seven years.

As part of my PhD, I spent some time trying to understand what factors influenced when and how women experience the menopause.

The first thing to highlight is there is not much research in this area and a lot more is needed. However, from what we do know, we know that different ethnic backgrounds, where you sit on the social ranks, as well as your medical history and lifestyle all influence when you transition into the menopause, the type of symptoms you experience and the severity of those symptoms.

Here is what I found:

1. The age your mother went through menopause used to be an indicator of when you would perhaps experience yours. However, as we now lead very different lives to those of our mothers, this isn't necessarily the case anymore. Add to this the fact that science has shown your genes control only about 10–15 per cent of your biology. Your environment controls the remainder, which is why what you eat and how you live are so powerful.

2. In the Western world, research shows that if you are overweight, smoke, drink alcohol regularly, are less active and eat ultra-processed foods, all this takes a toll on your hormones, potentially bringing menopause on earlier and increasing your chances of having hot flushes and night sweats.

3. The ethnic differences apparent in the research is interesting. Black and Hispanic women are more likely to experience the menopause earlier (by about two years). They have also been reported to be more likely to have severe menopausal symptoms and these symptoms have a higher chance of lasting longer. This may in part be linked to the social and health disparities we see across the board.

4. Stressful life events, IVF treatment, childbirth and extreme yo-yo dieting can also cause you to enter the menopause transition earlier. Women who have not had children or had them before the age of 28 will often go through an earlier perimenopause and menopause. Similarly, going through IVF cycles, which involves hyperstimulation of the ovaries, has been found to fast forward the road to perimenopause.

5. Smoking. We all know it's not good for us. Smokers reach menopause an average of two years earlier than non-smokers.

6. Medical history can also play a role. Women who are underweight or have low body fat will have lower overall oestrogen levels, which can lead to an earlier perimenopause. The opposite occurs in women with a higher body weight and more body fat (who are overweight or obese). Body fat produces a weak form of oestrogen, which means they are likely to have higher circulating levels overall and tend to go through the menopause later. However, this also means they have longer exposure to oestrogen, which comes with its own risks, like ovarian and womb cancer.

7. What we eat impacts our hormones. A typical Western diet that is high in refined carbohydrates, sugar, salt and man-made fat, and low in vegetables

and fruit, plays havoc with our hormones. A recent large study in the UK found that diets high in refined carbs were linked with earlier menopause, while a higher intake of oily fish and legumes was associated with a delayed onset of natural menopause (approximately 3.3 years per portion per day to be exact).

The duration and severity of symptoms also seems to depend on a variety of factors including when your first symptoms begin and your lifestyle. Research shows that the menopause journey can last anywhere from two to fourteen years but typically lasts around four to seven years.

Don't let all this dishearten or overwhelm you. Of course, none of us has just one attribute that will determine how and when our menopause journey plays out. It's always a complex interaction of factors that will play out differently in your own menopause journey. I am a sporty, working-class, mixed-race woman, not living in my country of origin, who experienced the stress of losing my father figure and my mum sixteen months apart, all while finishing my PhD, and I have not had children yet. You will have your own story. What I simply wanted to highlight is that there is no one formula to predict when you will begin your menopause journey and that is why it's important to know what to expect and to be proactive – and by reading this book you are well on your way. Yay! Go you!

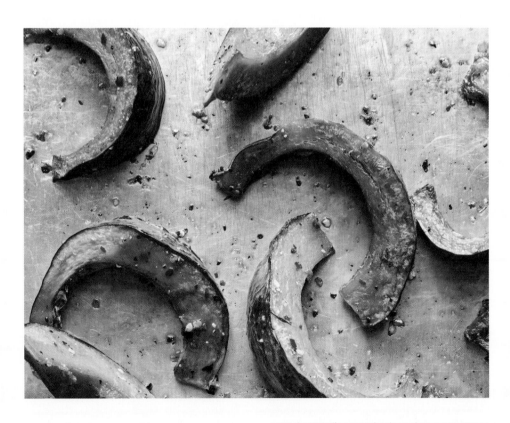

Perimenopause 101

A hormone flux does begin during this time, so it's important to understand what's going on. It's kinda like puberty but in reverse.

In a nutshell, a woman's ovaries reduce the amount of oestrogen and progesterone they produce over time. Our friend progesterone takes a dive first. She does so silently. Oestrogen also declines, but very often a little later in perimenopause. But for both, it's not necessarily a gentle glide down at this stage. For example, your progesterone levels may suddenly plummet, while your oestrogen levels remain erratically high. Fluctuating hormone levels become low hormone levels overall for both, and eventually they stop signalling to the ovaries to ovulate like clockwork, or to ovulate at all. No periods. Nada. Never again.

Perimenopause can be broken down into a few phases. Some experts break it down into four stages and others two. Let's keep it simple with two.

PHASE 1: EARLY PERIMENOPAUSE

While there is a big focus on oestrogen when we talk about hormonal issues, it's actually the fall in progesterone that very often drives the first symptoms we may experience. The first phase of the perimenopause is typically characterised by lowering progesterone levels and initially high-fluctuating levels of oestrogen. It is this unbalanced ratio between oestrogen and progesterone that can cause a lot of trouble and is the reason why some women find this phase more challenging than the latter stages of the menopause. A low progesterone-to-oestrogen balance is known as oestrogen dominance. Your menstrual cycle is likely to still be regular; however, as you have lower progesterone, it could be more sporadic. You are still able to have a baby in this phase.

PHASE 2: LATE PERIMENOPAUSE

During the early stage of this phase your cycle starts to become more irregular and can vary in length, sometimes by six to seven days. Hormone-wise, you continue to have low progesterone and high-fluctuating oestrogen. This means when oestrogen drops, it not only has further to fall but it can also drop to a lower level than what we are used to. Such a drop in oestrogen can trigger symptoms such as hot flushes and night sweats. As you progress through this stage, you start missing your periods and perhaps you have one cycle that is longer than sixty days. Your symptoms of high oestrogen actually start to ease as you begin to lose more oestrogen – even though it might still fluctuate. For example, your breast pain could ease, but night sweats and hot flushes could get worse. You can still fall pregnant in this phase.

Symptoms – messages from your body

Most women will experience symptoms at some point during their menopause transition, however the severity of symptoms varies widely. Some women don't experience symptoms severely enough to need attention or will only experience them for a few months. Others suffer for years – even decades. And in-between are a lot of women who don't feel like themselves but don't even think to link it to their hormones. They forge on with gritted teeth, thinking it's just life that is rubbish.

But symptoms are signals. If you have symptoms, then your hormones need some TLC. If perimenopause symptoms impact on your life, then you can seek support from your GP.

And you, my friend, have an active role to play in your own care. We call this self-management support. If you have more knowledge, you can direct the conversation, whether your healthcare professional is up on it or not. Knowledge is power, so it's time to get acquainted with some of the symptoms you may experience.

To help you navigate symptoms, I have split this section up a little. I have placed the ones you are most likely to experience in phase 1 into early perimenopause and those that are more characteristic of the later phase into late perimenopause. In reality, though, it isn't this clear-cut. There is massive overlap. Symptoms may come and go. Some may be subtle, while others can be full on. Some symptoms, like a dry vagina, might be easier to note – but generally feeling a bit off is harder to gauge. The key is to be aware and to begin a ritual of monthly check-ins as part of your self-care.

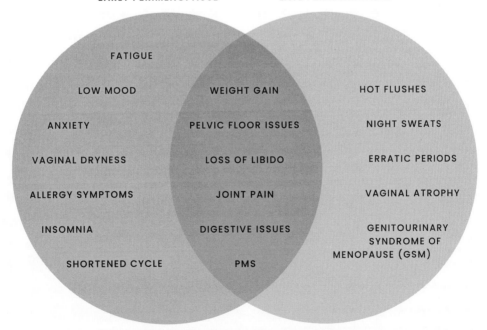

EARLY PERIMENOPAUSE

LATE PERIMENOPAUSE

FATIGUE

LOW MOOD

ANXIETY

VAGINAL DRYNESS

ALLERGY SYMPTOMS

INSOMNIA

SHORTENED CYCLE

WEIGHT GAIN

PELVIC FLOOR ISSUES

LOSS OF LIBIDO

JOINT PAIN

DIGESTIVE ISSUES

PMS

HOT FLUSHES

NIGHT SWEATS

ERRATIC PERIODS

VAGINAL ATROPHY

GENITOURINARY SYNDROME OF MENOPAUSE (GSM)

Symptoms of early perimenopause

While stress can be a challenge to manage at any age, it can be harder to cope with during your menopausal years.

LOW PROGESTERONE

Progesterone is the first hormone that takes a hit during perimenopause and a lot of the first symptoms we experience are linked to its decline. Progesterone is the cool, calm and collected hormone. It also helps us fall asleep, keeps oestrogen in check and protects us from the intense roller-coaster feelings that come with premenstrual syndrome (PMS). Hormones are complex, and everyone is a little different, but the most reported symptoms linked to low progesterone in this phase include:

> **Cycle changes:** Progesterone is the main hormone responsible for regulating your cycle. Changes to your normal cycle length could be due to low progesterone. You may experience heavier periods, longer periods, shorter cycles or irregular cycles.
> **Sleep changes:** Known as the 'relaxing hormone', progesterone has a mild sedative effect which means that low levels result in sleep difficulties, particularly in falling asleep.
> **Mood changes:** Progesterone is like a natural antidepressant. It has a calming effect on the brain as it stimulates the feel-good calming neurotransmitter GABA. Low progesterone is linked to feeling down, anxious and irritable. As you are likely to not be sleeping well, this may exacerbate the low mood and feelings of extreme PMS.
> **New allergy symptoms:** This is an ever evolving and currently widely debated area of nutrition, but what

we know is that women with low progesterone and high oestrogen are at increased risk of experiencing hayfever-type symptoms or the onset of new allergies due to an intolerance to histamine. Histamine is a natural substance found in our bodies and in some foods. It has many functions in the body, including supporting our immune system and digestion, and plays an important role in communicating messages to your brain. Histamine intolerance means that you have a high level of histamine in your body. This can happen if your body cannot break down histamine. Progesterone, which helps to stabilise mast cells (the cells responsible for histamine release) decreases in this stage, potentially increasing histamine-related symptoms. Oestrogen enhances histamine release, making the body prone to histamine accumulation. While symptoms vary from person to person, some common reactions include excessive bloating, skin rashes, coughing, migraines and brain fog.

LOW PROGESTERONE SIGNS
- *Suddenly everything and anything irritates you. You need more time alone.*
- *Your cycles may be shorter and your periods heavier than usual.*
- *Headaches before your cycle.*
- *Trouble falling asleep.*

THE STRESS–PROGESTERONE LINK

Modern-day living is full of pressure and stress – getting too little sleep, taking care of kids, hustling to pay off that ever-increasing mortgage while dealing with aging parents that behave like children and, in the middle of it all, needing to find some time to take the cat to the vet. What's more, science suggests that stress in all forms is cumulative. Unresolved trauma, physical, mental or emotional, can cause our nervous systems to always be on high alert. Over time, this trauma is often normalised or suppressed through coping strategies like comfort eating, alcohol, drugs or an online shopping addiction. If it's not dealt with, your body keeps score.

Combine all this with the big hormonal shift of perimenopause and it is the perfect storm. While stress can be a challenge to manage at any age, it can be harder to cope with during your menopausal years. The menopause transition is a naturally occurring stress on the body, so baseline levels of the stress hormone cortisol may be higher throughout this time. Cortisol is also essentially made from the same precursor molecule as progesterone, so when the demands to make more cortisol increase, the body prioritises survival over reproduction and progesterone loses out. This is termed the 'pregnenolone steal'.

In addition to this, during the menopause transition, the adrenal glands are meant to take over some of the work of the diminishing ovaries and produce small amounts of progesterone and oestrogen. However, the adrenal glands cannot produce these hormones efficiently when they are pumping out stress hormones. This means there is even less progesterone.

It's a bit like dominoes. Less progesterone means an even lower progesterone–oestrogen ratio, which means oestrogen becomes excessive and troublemaker mode is activated (i.e. oestrogen dominance).

When we have optimal progesterone levels, our body can buffer stress. Once

THE IMPACT OF CHRONICALLY ELEVATED CORTISOL

- Frequent colds and feeling run-down.
- Low energy, even if you are getting enough rest.
- Craving foods that are high in sugar and fat.
- Digestion problems like bloating.
- Insomnia or frequent waking.
- Weight gain, especially around the middle.
- Low sex drive.
- Reduced liver function (i.e. feeling generally unwell).
- Inflammation: High doses of cortisone medication can reduce inflammation, but over time, chronically high levels of cortisol increase inflammation and the risk of diseases like diabetes and dementia.

Taking care of yourself has never been more of a priority.

these levels start to lower during perimenopause, the cortisol-buffering effect weakens. Higher cortisol means lower DHEA. If your cortisol/DHEA ratio is out, this will compromise every other hormone ratio. Any symptoms you may be experiencing are exacerbated a gazillion times. It sounds dramatic, I know, but, ladies, this is an important message: your forty-year-old self needs to learn to manage her stress now more than ever before. If there is one thing you take away from this, let it be that taking care of yourself has never been more of a priority.

OESTROGEN DOMINANCE

While the menopause sees a decrease in both our female hormones, oestrogen and progesterone, over time, a lot of the symptoms experienced, particularly in the first phase of perimenopause, are caused by – wait for it – too much oestrogen!

There are two main reasons why you can end up with too much oestrogen (oestrogen dominance). Firstly, the ratio of oestrogen to progesterone is thrown out during perimenopause. If you cast your mind back to page 15, you'll recall that progesterone and oestrogen are like BFFs that work together to keep the body in balance. They both play a role in fertility, mood, vitality and overall wellbeing. In excess, oestrogen tends to have a more aggressive effect on the body compared with progesterone, which is more calming. At 35, a woman's oestrogen-to-progesterone ratio is balanced. As a woman approaches her forties, progesterone can begin to drop a lot faster compared with oestrogen, which then creates an imbalance where oestrogen becomes dominant.

Another reason why you can end up with too much oestrogen is if there is an issue with breaking it down. There are two places where this breaking down occurs: the liver and the gut.

The liver story

When I was in my twenties, I could be on the shots of tequila, go to bed, get up, go for a run and then go to lectures and be functional. Now, if I try to have even one tequila, when I wake up, I feel like I need a whole week in bed! As you age, your liver isn't as efficient and effective as it once was. This doesn't just apply to alcohol but to the metabolism of hormones as well. This can create a challenge for us in our forties as we need our liver to be in good form. It is responsible for breaking down different types of oestrogen into smaller pieces as the first step in the process of eliminating metabolised oestrogen.

If your liver is already overloaded or is not in tiptop condition, it does a bit of a slapdash job at breaking down oestrogens to eliminate them properly.

The gut story

Gut health is a bit of a trendy term at the moment. Inside your body is an ecosystem of trillions of microorganisms (bacteria, viruses and fungi). Known as your microbiota, this collection of microorganisms not only helps you digest food, it helps to regulate your metabolism, your hormones and your mood. It affects the strength of your immune system and your risk of diseases. Basically, there isn't much going on in your body (and mind) that isn't influenced by the composition of your microbiome. A healthy gut means a healthy body and mind.

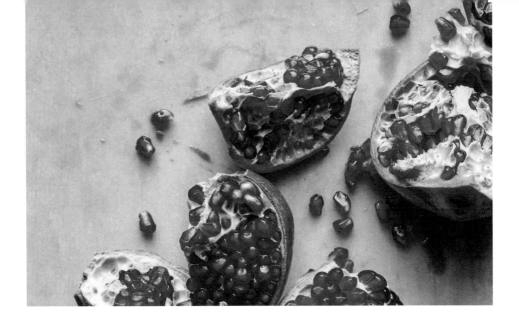

Only in recent years has science begun to really appreciate the importance of the human microbiome and how our internal ecosystem works. A healthy microbiome is made up of both 'good' and 'bad' microorganisms, in the right amounts and located in the right places, working together to create a vibrant ecosystem that works in harmony. But if there is a disturbance in that balance – brought on by the prolonged use of antibiotics, or other bacteria-destroying medication, or a poor diet and unhealthy lifestyle – dysbiosis can occur (an imbalance in good and bad bacteria that may affect your gut lining). As a result of this imbalance, the body becomes more susceptible to disease. While there is no 'optimal' microbiome that indicates whether someone is healthy or not, what we do know is that having lots of different bacterial species is good. This is called microbial diversity.

Within your microbiome is a subset of microbes called the estrobolome that impact the metabolism and the balance of the various forms of hormones, but particularly oestrogen. I mean, how brilliant are our bodies?

You have an entire microbiome department dedicated to the task of regulating your oestrogen levels.

When this system is working, you absorb and excrete the right balance of oestrogen. It's a win-win situation. Healthy oestrogen levels in turn support a healthy gut, as oestrogen maintains the integrity of your gut lining. If your oestrogen levels are out of whack, this has a knock-on effect of gut permeability, known as 'leaky' gut. The concept of gut permeability is evolving, however, very simply put, research suggests that increased gut permeability means trouble. The dysbiosis can lead to either a deficiency or an excess of free oestrogen and an imbalance between the various forms of oestrogens and other hormones.

Oestrogen dominance experienced in menopause can adversely affect the estrobolome, as can other factors such as stress, lack of sleep, smoking, inactivity, diets high in added sugar and ultra-processed foods and overuse of antibiotics and other medications.

HIGH-OESTROGEN SYMPTOMS

Symptoms of oestrogen dominance vary from person to person and depend largely on the severity of the hormonal imbalance. See the diagram opposite for an overview of the symptoms you may experience. Of these, I want to highlight some of the ones I commonly see in my clinic.

Irregular periods

In a healthy body, oestrogen and progesterone naturally balance each other out. Having oestrogen dominance can lead to an overgrowth of the lining of the uterus (endometrium), which in turn causes heavy periods. Your periods can become closer together or more irregular. Women with a fluctuation in oestrogen levels are more likely to experience irregular periods. Fluctuating periods are often the first indication of perimenopause. They may get lighter or heavier, change their duration or be missed entirely.

Weight gain

Weight gain can be a trigger for many people. While it's not an inevitable symptom of the menopause transition, it is the one that is most visible. A lot of people come to see me with weight gain or lack of weight loss as a pain point. A combination of hormone changes, fatigue and stress-induced comfort eating means it is quite common to gain some weight during perimenopause. The statistics say that on average, women in the perimenopause gain about 5 pounds (2.2 kilograms). The way the body stores fat also changes. A telltale sign that you may be having issues with your oestrogen levels is weight gain, particularly around the middle. In earlier years, weight gain is around the hips and thighs, but with perimenopause it becomes more concentrated around the middle. As our ovaries produce less oestrogen, the body starts to look for it elsewhere. Fat cells also produce oestrogen, so the body tries to create more of this oestrogen by building up fat stores. Low testosterone also means our metabolism slows down due to lower muscle mass. Menopausal women also metabolise carbohydrates differently, which means they are more likely to become insulin resistant.

Low mood

Let's be honest – changes to our mental health have a knock-on effect on pretty much every aspect of life. It can be disturbing to find yourself feeling uncharacteristically nervous, depressed or having memory lapses. Sometimes these feelings can even strain your relationships with others. It helps to know that the psychological effects of menopause are temporary. Hormone shifts affect mood. With increased levels of oestrogen, you may experience extreme emotions as oestrogen affects the way chemical messengers send signals throughout the brain. Fluctuating levels of progesterone and testosterone can aggravate low mood, feelings of irritability and even extreme anger. This can happen in the lead-up to and/or the aftermath of your period.

Poor memory and concentration

Some women find that perimenopause brings occasional memory lapses, often related to reduced ability to concentrate. Brain fog is a collective term given to symptoms that encompass poor concentration, poor memory and a general 'fuzzy' feeling.

Oestrogen does a lot for the brain. It stimulates the brain cells to take up glucose and produce energy so they work efficiently. It also works with neurotransmitters to send signals to the brain's memory and emotional centre, which means that when oestrogen levels ebb and flow, it can affect our memory, concentration and emotional wellbeing. Other symptoms, such as fatigue and poor sleep, can also make brain fog worse.

Digestive issues

Hormonal changes in perimenopause affect our gut and the amount of acid in our stomach and slow down digestion. Bloating is a common symptom caused by the hormonal shifts. Higher oestrogen can also cause water retention, which can exacerbate the bloat.

During this phase, you continue to experience low levels of progesterone and high-fluctuating oestrogen. The ongoing impact of these hormone changes most commonly shows up in the following symptoms.

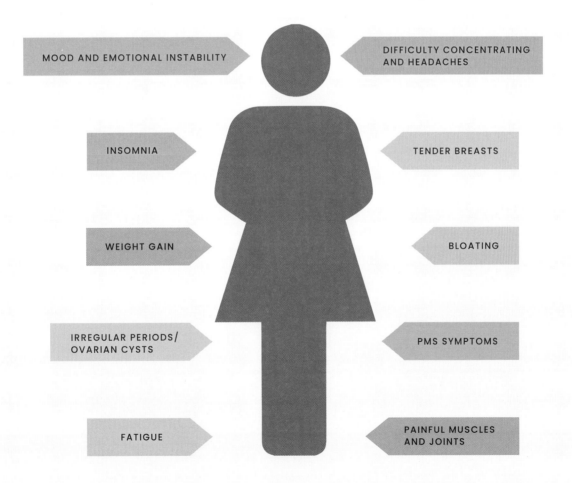

MOOD AND EMOTIONAL INSTABILITY

DIFFICULTY CONCENTRATING AND HEADACHES

INSOMNIA

TENDER BREASTS

WEIGHT GAIN

BLOATING

IRREGULAR PERIODS/ OVARIAN CYSTS

PMS SYMPTOMS

FATIGUE

PAINFUL MUSCLES AND JOINTS

Symptoms of late perimenopause

During this phase, you continue to experience low levels of progesterone and high-fluctuating oestrogen. The ongoing impact of these hormone changes most commonly shows up in the following symptoms.

HOT FLUSHES

Hot flushes are the classic menopause symptom and the most common one, affecting 75 per cent of women. They come on suddenly at any time of the day and spread throughout the face, chest and body. They may be accompanied by other symptoms like sweating, dizziness or even heart palpations. The exact reason why they occur is not known. Some believe it's due to falling oestrogen levels, which then affect another hormone, noradrenaline, which regulates our body temperature. But oestrogen also directly affects the thermoregulatory areas of our brains. There is no 'normal' number of hot flushes. It's individual.

NIGHT SWEATS

Night sweats, as the name indicates, are hot flushes that strike at night. They are often the main reason why many women struggle with sleep, as they wake up drenched in sweat and have to change the sheets.

VAGINAL HEALTH

Vaginal issues affect 80 per cent of women but very few talk about it. Oestrogen keeps your vagina healthy by acting as a natural lubricant. Lower levels of oestrogen may cause the tissues of the vulva and the lining of the vagina to become thinner and less elastic, which may result in dryness, itchiness and inflammation. The natural bacterial community (the vaginal microbiome) is also affected by the decline in oestrogen, with the bacterial species, in particular lactobacillus, declining. Reduced levels of oestrogen also result in changes in the pH balance of the vagina, making it less acidic and more alkaline, which can increase the likelihood of vaginal and urinary infections. Sex may be painful, and normal everyday activities, such as riding a bike or walking, can be uncomfortable.

SKIN CHANGES

During this phase, women often complain that their skin feels tight and dry and looks dull. Fine lines appear more prominent and some women see the return of acne from their younger years. Oestrogen helps keep our skin lubricated; it gives skin its fullness and reduces fine lines and dryness. It also helps build collagen, which is a protein that gives our skin structure and strength. Collagen begins to decline as early as your twenties. So, when you reach your forties, your collagen production is almost cut in half.

PAINFUL MUSCLES AND JOINTS

Oestrogen is important in providing lubrication for your joints and preventing inflammation, so an oestrogen deficiency can cause aches and pains in your joints. Collagen is also a vital component of bones, joints and cartilage, so lower levels also lead to joint pain and stiffness.

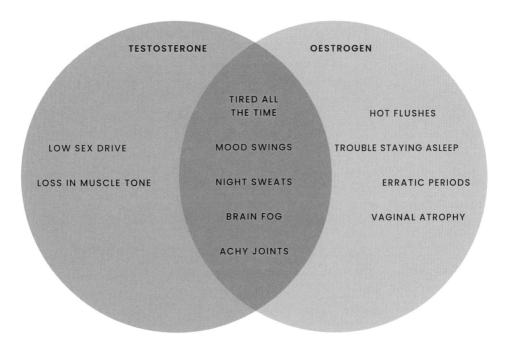

TESTOSTERONE

OESTROGEN

TIRED ALL
THE TIME

LOW SEX DRIVE

MOOD SWINGS

HOT FLUSHES

TROUBLE STAYING ASLEEP

LOSS IN MUSCLE TONE

NIGHT SWEATS

ERRATIC PERIODS

BRAIN FOG

VAGINAL ATROPHY

ACHY JOINTS

WHERE DOES TESTOSTERONE FIT IN?

Between our twenties and forties, our testosterone levels decline by approximately 50 per cent. This means that some of the first symptoms of the perimenopause – feeling tired all the time, lower-quality sleep, reduced libido and loss of lean muscle – are often caused by decreasing testosterone levels. Later on in the perimenopause, low testosterone may also impact night sweats. Above is a snapshot that can help you understand which symptoms are linked with which hormones. However, do keep in mind this is an over-simplification, so it should serve purely as a guide.

BE SYMPTOM SAVVY

The tricky thing about the perimenopause is there is no clear-cut test you can do to tell you whether you are in it or not. Hormone blood tests vary so much during your perimenopausal years that they are not always beneficial. A key part of diagnosing the perimenopause is to be symptom savvy.

It really helps to have a detailed account of what you think your 'normal' is so that you can be cognisant of any changes that occur. Keep a log of all the symptoms you are experiencing so you can see how things may be changing over time and pick up any patterns and pain points. I would suggest that you make this symptom check-in a part of your self-care. You can use my symptom checker on page 250, or the UK-based Menopause Charity has a useful online tool.

When you see your health professional, make a list of the questions you wish to discuss to ensure they understand your agenda from the start, and will cover the things that are most important to you.

Postmenopausal health

Now's the time to focus on heart, bone and brain health.

The effects of reduced oestrogen can also have a long-term impact on our health as we move into the postmenopausal phase. This is the time after you've been without a menstrual period for twelve months. Classic menopausal symptoms, such as hot flushes, may get milder or go away, but now's the time to focus on heart, bone and brain health.

YOUR HEART

Many women think that heart disease is a man's disease but it isn't. Heart disease is the number one killer of women. In fact, after the age of fifty, nearly half of all deaths in women are due to some form of cardiovascular disease. Once women reach the age of fifty, the age of natural menopause, their risk of heart disease increases dramatically.

In the short term, the hormonal fluctuations can cause heart palpitations (a sensation where your heart is beating faster than normal). This can also happen in a hot flush. In the longer term, our risk of cardiovascular disease increases, as oestrogen helps to protect our arteries by reducing the build-up of fatty plaques that can cause the arteries to narrow. When the arteries narrow, blood and oxygen can't reach your vital organs. Low oestrogen can also cause your cholesterol numbers to go up, increase your blood pressure and raise the inflammatory level in your body.

YOUR BONES

Around 10 per cent of a woman's bone mass is lost in the first five years of the menopause and this increases your risk of osteoporosis, a condition that affects your bones so they become weaker and are more likely to break. This is because oestrogen helps to keep your bones strong and healthy. Less oestrogen puts you at risk of developing osteoporosis. While we may not be able to travel back in time, we can preserve and strengthen the bones we have. Muscles and bones are also intricately linked, so you need to strengthen your muscles too as this supports your bones.

YOUR BRAIN

Alzheimer's disease is the most common type of dementia, affecting between 60–70 per cent of people with dementia. Approximately two-thirds of people diagnosed with Alzheimer's disease are women. Alzheimer's is more common in women after menopause. Studies indicate that women who went through menopause prematurely or before the age of forty are at the greatest risk, which supports the notion that oestrogen has a protective role in brain health that may be lost when levels decrease. Research in rats shows that a reduction in oestrogen makes the brain more prone to learning and memory problems, both of which are related to Alzheimer's disease.

How to adapt to changing hormones

There are many treatment options available to support you through the menopause, so you don't need to suffer in silence. You may opt for medical management through hormone replacement therapy (HRT) or not – either way, addressing your lifestyle is pivotal, as it will be a formidable ally in your menopause journey. Remember, no two of us are the same; it is about finding out what works and feels right for you. Be proactive – don't wait until your symptoms become unmanageable before you seek support. Begin the conversation; talk to a health professional about the options available to you.

Hormone replacement therapy (HRT)

For the following section I asked two medical colleagues to answer some frequently asked questions about HRT. Dr Elise Dallas is a General Practitioner at The London General Practice and specialises in menopausal care. Dr Adam Carey is a doctor and leading commentator on all areas of sports nutrition and human performance.

1. WHAT IS HRT?

Dr Elise says: 'Hormone replacement therapy (HRT) is supplementing women with one or more of the hormones oestrogen, progesterone and testosterone that are lost during the menopausal transition. These are hormones already made by your body in your ovaries. HRT is recommended by national guidelines as the first choice for women who have symptoms caused by low or fluctuating hormone levels. It has been shown to offer the most effective relief from symptoms, and for the majority of women, the benefits of taking HRT outweigh the risks.'

2. WHO SHOULDN'T TAKE HRT?

Dr Adam says: 'Interestingly there are almost no absolute contraindications to taking oestrogen-based HRT and every woman should be assessed based on their needs. If a woman has ever had a reproductive cancer like breast, uterine or ovarian, where the oestrogen might encourage the growth of cancerous cells, this needs to be discussed with their doctor before considering HRT. However, in women where one of these tumours has been treated, oestrogen therapy can still be used under medical supervision from a menopause specialist, if it is felt that the benefits outweigh the potential risks. Similarly, women with a strong family history of breast and ovarian cancers may not be such good candidates for HRT but should not be excluded from consideration. Smokers and those with abnormal liver function also need careful consideration by a clinical team.'

3. WHEN SHOULD YOU BEGIN TAKING HRT?

Dr Elise says: 'It is best to start taking HRT when you start to experience symptoms that have any negative impact on your quality of life. For many women, these symptoms emerge

Our hormones are influenced by how we live and what we eat. Our lifestyle matters.

during perimenopause, the period leading up to menopause. You do not need to wait until your periods have stopped to start taking HRT. HRT is recommended as first-line treatment for managing the symptoms, and for the majority of women who start taking HRT before the age of sixty, the benefits of taking it outweigh the risks.

'While the most significant long-term health benefits are observed in women who commence HRT within ten years of menopause, HRT can be initiated at any age. There is limited research on the advantages of starting HRT in older women, as this area has not been extensively studied. Nonetheless, most healthy women can still derive benefits from HRT, even if it has been more than a decade since their menopause. This decision should be made on an individual basis.'

4. IS THERE ANY TIME TO STOP TAKING HRT?

Dr Elise says: 'According to guidance from the British Menopause Society, there is no strict limit to the duration of HRT use. If you continue to be healthy and feel the benefits of taking HRT, there is no reason to stop. The decision to continue treatment should be based on your specific circumstances. The dosage, treatment plan and duration of HRT should be tailored to your individual needs, with an annual assessment of the advantages and disadvantages of ongoing HRT use. In cases of early menopause or ovarian removal surgery, the timing is calculated from the age of fifty, which is the average age for menopause.

'For older women, lower oestrogen doses are often suitable, and the safest way to take replacement oestrogen is through the skin, administered through patches, gels or sprays. Even a small amount of replacement oestrogen can effectively address symptoms and offer essential bone and heart protection. If you have a uterus, adding a progestogen, like micronised progesterone, is necessary to protect the lining of the uterus.'

5. WHAT BLOOD TESTS ARE AVAILABLE?

Dr Adam says: 'If you are over the age of 45, most women do not need a blood test to diagnose their menopausal symptoms and treatment is usually based on reported symptoms. If you get symptoms before the age of forty, this is called a premature menopause or primary ovarian insufficiency. This will be investigated with blood tests to look at both your pituitary function and production of luteinising hormone (LH) and follicle-stimulating hormone (FSH), together with levels of the steroid hormones, oestrogen, progesterone and testosterone.'

6. WHAT ARE THE HRT ALTERNATIVES?

Dr Adam says: 'There are many alternative and complementary therapies that may provide benefits, both for the classic symptoms of the menopause, but also bone and muscle strength, mood and cognitive function.

'There are also a number of other, non-hormonal drugs that doctors can use to treat vasomotor symptoms that impact on mood. These include clonidine, gabapentin and selective serotonin reuptake inhibitors (SSRIs).'

See opposite for alternatives to HRT.

ALTERNATIVE AND COMPLEMENTARY THERAPIES

Dr Adam says:

- *'Alternative therapies, such as acupuncture and acupressure, can be useful, although the evidence from good studies is lacking and more research in these areas is needed. If you're considering them, they should be provided by a qualified professional.*
- *'Herbal treatments have been studied and their benefits have been identified, however clinical guidelines recommend using products that have been licensed or carry the traditional herbal registration (THR) number or the equivalent in your country. It's important to recognise that some of these treatments may interact with other medicines and their use should be discussed with your healthcare professional.*
- *'Cognitive behavioural therapy (CBT) programs have been found to be useful not only for helping to reduce anxiety and improve the mood disturbances women may experience, but they have also been shown to reduce hot flushes and night sweats. These techniques can also help improve sleep that is often disturbed by menopausal symptoms. There are self-help courses available which have been shown to have a positive impact.'*

Lifestyle treatments

Our hormones are influenced by how we live and what we eat. Our lifestyle matters. Whether or not you choose to take HRT, tweaking your lifestyle will make a difference. There are some things we can all do to make for a smoother transition to the menopause. The rest of this book will focus on the management of the menopause transition through a holistic lifestyle, focusing mainly on what you eat.

CALL TO ACTION

Step 1: Track your cycle. No matter your age. This is a must. There are so many apps out there. Try Flo, Clue or Wild AI.

Step 2: Adopt a symptom stocktake ritual. You can begin this at any age but in your forties you should prioritise it as part of your self-care. Sit down and check in with yourself. How are you? Are there any changes? Use the symptom checker (see page 250) to help.

Step 3: Know your baseline. Get a hormone profile test. If you are still in your thirties, get your baseline hormones tested as that is the best time to do it. If you are already in your forties and didn't do it in your thirties, the second-best time is now! Granted, in some countries, this is a harder one to action. Under the National Health Service in the UK, for example, baseline bloods would not be done if there were no symptoms. This emphasises the importance of Step 2 and noticing your symptoms. Numbers from blood tests should never be used in isolation. Symptoms matter. Know yours. Track yours.

PART 2

Eating for success

The four key nutrition principles

In the previous chapter I wanted you to notice and record any changes, so you can use your symptoms as tools to learn more about yourself. In this chapter, I'll lay the foundations for nourishing your body and teach you how to eat to make your hormones work for you, not against you. While you're in the menopause transition you might feel as though your body is all over the place but you actually do have control over your mindset, your lifestyle and your environment – all of which affect the symptoms that go along with menopause.

Healthy eating is not a replacement for hormone therapy (should you choose to have it), however nutrition is a formidable ally. Similarly, going on HRT does not mean you don't need to address your lifestyle. Lifestyle matters. It can help you feel and function better, it can support the management of your symptoms and it is fundamental to prepping you for the menopause. In this chapter, I'll introduce you to the four key nutrition principles for optimal hormone balance:

> optimal hydration
> controlled blood-sugar levels
> a healthy gut microbiome
> anti-inflammatory eating.

I'll show you what you should be putting on your plate to help calm your hormones, improve your energy, reduce your cravings, keep your waistline in check and, in the long term, keep your heart, brain, bones and joints healthy.

I won't be offering you any 'quick fixes' or selling radical measures. My approach is centred around balance. It's about nailing the basics most of the time to establish good hormonal balance and symptom management. Then I will teach you how to add layers of icing and chocolate sprinkles that can take it up a level, should you want that. But the first thing is to have a good cake base – metaphorically speaking! Ready?

DISCLAIMER
The world we live in loves a magic, cure-all solution. If only it was so easy! We are all different; our genes, physiology, gut bacteria, tastebuds, previous traumas and personal circumstances make each of us unique. My job is to help people become their healthiest, strongest, best-performing selves – in a way that works for their lives and bodies. In my fifteen-plus years of working with clients I have learned a few things.

> Different people have different responses. One size doesn't fit all.
> An all-or-nothing approach doesn't work for most people.
> Nutritional habits that are successful feel reasonable, enjoyable and sustainable.
> Sustainablity is everything – create habits and eating plans you can stick to in the long term.

Principle 1: Hydration

Low energy, a 4pm slump, headaches, mood swings, brain fog, urinary tract infections on repeat and dry skin. They sound like some of the menopausal symptoms we talked about in chapter 1, right? They could be. But they are also symptoms people commonly report when they don't drink enough water.

You may be thinking: just drink more water? Is that it? And that is exactly the point. We all know that water is good for us but many people underestimate the powerful role it plays in our bodies and brains.

Your entire body is 75 per cent water and 80 per cent of your brain composition is water. Water transports nutrients that allow your body to generate energy. It gives your tissues and cells their form. It keeps your heart pumping. It helps your brain send messages effectively. It helps you to remember things. It lubricates your joints. It keeps your gut working like clockwork. It's linked with how hungry or full you feel.

WHAT HAPPENS WHEN YOU'RE DEHYDRATED

While most people never experience severe dehydration, a large majority go through life in a state of chronic mild dehydration. In order to get on top of your hormones, you need to tackle this. Being dehydrated happens when you lose more water than you take in. Mild dehydration occurs when you experience a water loss of 1–2 per cent. Practically speaking, when you are thirsty, you are mildly dehydrated.

At this point, research shows that your brain shrinks and you begin to suffer cognitive side effects such as poor memory and lower concentration and mood. New research using MRIs suggests that when a brain is dehydrated, the aging linked to dementia is accelerated. Yikes! If I needed a cue to reach for my water bottle, this is it.

Regularly drinking enough water can help you have more energy, improve your digestion, increase your concentration and memory and help regulate your appetite. In a recent study, dieters who drank 500 millilitres of water half an hour before meals lost almost twice as much weight over a 12-week period as those who didn't drink the water. The thinking behind this is that drinking water before a meal makes you feel fuller, so as a result, you eat less during your meal.

In addition, when you don't drink enough day to day, your energy levels dip and you feel tired. When you feel tired, your body starts to confuse thirst with a need to eat to boost your energy levels, so you feel hungry. If you're already struggling with your weight, it's not an ideal scenario.

Exercise also feels harder when you are mildly dehydrated. Your muscles cramp more, you will feel more bloated and retain more water. We already know that our hormones can give us a hard time during the menopause, so why would you want to exacerbate your symptoms by becoming dehydrated?

Simply drinking more water could be one of the healthiest changes you make.

OBSTACLES

Simply drinking more water could be one of the healthiest changes you make. But I get it; it can be a hard habit to crack. There are often a multitude of obstacles in our way preventing us from being well hydrated. These might include the following.

> **Weaker bladder control:** Lower levels of oestrogen in the menopause can cause thinning of the urethra and consequent symptoms of leakage of urine with coughing, laughing, sneezing or lifting objects, which can be embarrassing. It can also cause you to have an 'overactive bladder', which gives you a sudden urge to urinate. If you are experiencing these symptoms, you may have dialled down your water intake as a result.
> **You forget:** Many of us struggle to fit it all in. This includes remembering to drink water. You may go through the day from one cup of tea or coffee to the next, and by the time you get home after a day of work, you realise you have not drunk much water, so you glug down one glass between chores in the evening.
> **You don't have time:** You are already time poor. You don't want to be 'wasting' time taking countless toilet breaks.
> **The taste:** Water isn't exactly the most delicious, tasty thing out there. If it was sweetened with a little something, it would be more appealing, right?

If these resonate with you, it's okay – you're not alone, but it is time to make some changes.

HYDRATION HACKS

Establish a routine

The amount of water each person needs every day varies. We get an estimated 20 per cent of our hydration needs from food like veggies and fruit. As a guide, you should drink 1.5–2 litres of water a day. If you're active, it's hotter or you are a heavier sweater, you will need more! Make it a habit. I am a big fan of using a water bottle to track my water intake over the day. Checking the colour of your urine is also a good way to keep on top of your hydration. Apart from the first urination of the day, your urine should be a pale straw colour. It shouldn't change the colour of the water in the toilet bowl too much. If it's darker than that, you need to drink more water. The exception is if you are taking B vitamins as this will colour your urine, making it a brighter yellow.

Get in there early

Water is vital for performance, so we need to ensure that we are staying hydrated during the day. Try to drink most of your fluids earlier in the day. Ideally, you should have drunk the majority of your fluids by 6pm and what you drink in the evening should be purely for pleasure. If you drink too much fluid in the evening, you will also end up needing a loo run in the night, which is less than ideal. Waking up to go to the loo in the middle of the night shouldn't be happening routinely. If you have to go, don't turn the lights on if you can avoid it, to minimise the impact on your sleep (more on this on page 83).

Make water fun

You don't need to buy expensive bottled water. Using a simple water filter can help reduce the taste of chlorine that some water has. If you need to make your water more interesting, add pieces of lemon, orange, mint or cucumber. I'm not a fan of routinely drinking cordials – even if they are low sugar (more on that on page 65). Personally, I like room-temperature water, although cold water can help lower your temperature after a hard workout. Herbal tea and non-caffeinated options count towards your fluid intake, too.

Train your bladder

As you drink more water, you don't need to be peeing all the time. If you find that you are always going to the loo, then you have set your bladder 'thermostat' at a very low volume and you need to reset it to a higher volume. When you get the urge to go, try to hold it for an extra five minutes before going to the bathroom. Each week, add five more minutes to the time you hold the urine after you have the urge. The goal is to urinate every two to four hours during the day, and hold about a pint (300–400ml) between toilet breaks.

Train your pelvic floor muscles

You don't need to endure problems with urinary incontinence. Exercises to train and strengthen the pelvic floor muscles may help. You can also speak to your doctor about other options.

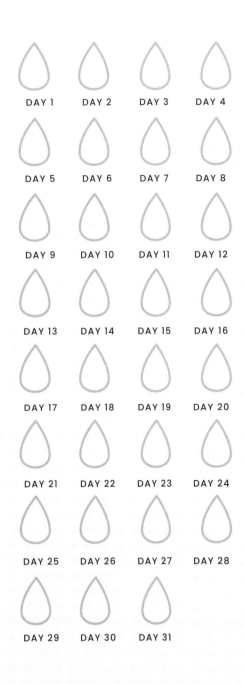

BOTTOMS-UP CHALLENGE MONTH

Try to drink 2 litres of water a day for a whole month. Use this chart to tick off each day as you complete it.

DAY 1   DAY 2   DAY 3   DAY 4

DAY 5   DAY 6   DAY 7   DAY 8

DAY 9   DAY 10   DAY 11   DAY 12

DAY 13   DAY 14   DAY 15   DAY 16

DAY 17   DAY 18   DAY 19   DAY 20

DAY 21   DAY 22   DAY 23   DAY 24

DAY 25   DAY 26   DAY 27   DAY 28

DAY 29   DAY 30   DAY 31

COFFEE AND THE MENOPAUSE

If you find it hard to imagine mornings without a coffee, you might be wondering how it might affect you during the menopause. Caffeine is a stimulant and for some people, it can take up to ten hours to completely clear from the bloodstream. A recent study of 2507 menopausal women found that those with a higher caffeine intake were more likely to have hot flushes and night sweats – however, they were also likely to have fewer problems with mood, memory and concentration. We all respond differently to caffeine based on our genetic make-up. If you enjoy coffee and can tolerate its caffeine content, then you can keep your coffee habit (within the recommended levels). However, if you don't tolerate caffeine well and struggle with hot flushes, ease up on the caffeine, and be sure to have your last caffeinated drink by 2pm.

Caffeine recommendations

Daily caffeine limits:

> Pregnant women: 200mg a day
> Everyone else: 400mg a day.

Typical beverages contain:

> 1 mug (220ml) instant coffee (one teaspoon): 30–35mg caffeine
> 1 mug (200ml) filter coffee: 90–140mg caffeine
> Double espresso shot (60ml x2): 125–160mg caffeine
> 1 cup (220ml) tea: 40–50mg caffeine
> 1 cup (220ml) green tea*: 30–35mg caffeine
> 30g dark chocolate: 20–40mg caffeine.

*Green tea contains less caffeine than black, but also has higher levels of an amino acid called L-theanine, which calms the nervous system.

TAKEAWAYS

1. Optimal hydration is fundamental to good health. Mild dehydration exacerbates menopause symptoms such as low energy, moodiness, irritability, gut issues, a craving for sweet stuff and hot flushes.

2. Simply drinking more water could be one of the healthiest changes you can make to support your body.

3. The amount of water that a person needs every day varies. As a guide, drink 1.5 to 2 litres of water a day. If you're active, or it's hotter or you are a heavier sweater, you will need more! Drink most of your water earlier in the day. Make it a habit.

4. Water is the best choice of drink. Flavour it with pieces of fruit or mint for variety. Herbal teas can be included in your fluid intake as well.

5. Checking the colour of your urine is a good self-feedback mechanism you can use day to day to keep on top of your hydration. Apart from the first urination of the day, your urine should be a pale straw colour.

Principle 2: Controlling blood-sugar levels

Blood-sugar (also called blood-glucose) control is one of the nutritional areas I coach every single client on. It is the backbone of healthy eating, the cornerstone of mental and physical performance. Learn to manage your blood-sugar levels and your world will feel better. Your energy, your mood, your focus, your cravings, your waistline, your sleep, your va-va-voom, your risk of chronic diseases in the future and, of course, your hormones, will all benefit. You don't need to become obsessed with your blood sugar, but you do need to take note of it.

Managing your blood-sugar levels is important at any stage of life, but even more so when your oestrogen levels are decreasing, as they are in the menopause. Research has shown that our friend oestrogen plays an important role in affecting the way your body responds to insulin. Insulin is the key hormone linked to blood-sugar control. Less oestrogen means we are predisposed to poor blood-glucose control if we are not on top of it.

In order to nail blood-sugar control, we need to understand the three main macronutrients in our diet: carbohydrates, proteins and fats.

WHAT ARE CARBOHYDRATES?

Carbohydrates are our main source of energy. When most people think of carbs, they generally think about the starchy carbs: bread, pasta, rice, potatoes, for example. What they forget is that vegetables, fruit and legumes are carbs too.

Carbohydrates are essentially sugar molecules bonded together to varying degrees. Broadly speaking, there are two types of carbohydrates: refined and unrefined.

Refined carbohydrates

Refined carbs are man-modified plant foods, industrially processed to improve their shelf life, taste and texture. This means they tend to come with additives, emulsifiers and preservatives. Think about those crunchy potato chips or that milk chocolate that melts perfectly in the mouth. Processing significantly changes the way the food is digested and absorbed, typically increasing the rate at which it is digested, which often means an increased rate of absorption of the food's sugars. Within this category you also have small molecules known as monosaccharides and disaccharides that need very little digestion at all. These are called 'free sugars' or added sugar.

Refined carbs include the following:

> white bread and other items made with white flour, like pastries and cakes
> chocolate and confectionery
> sugar-sweetened drinks
> many breakfast cereals
> flavoured yoghurt.

The sugars found in honey, syrups (such as maple and golden), unsweetened fruit juices, vegetable juices and smoothies all occur naturally, but still count as free sugars. (The sugar that's found naturally in milk, whole fruit and vegetables does not count as free sugars.)

Unrefined (complex) carbohydrates

Unrefined carbs, on the other hand, are more complex in structure and therefore need more digestion. Complex carbohydrates include starchy carbohydrates and fibrous carbohydrates. The sugar molecules in starch are bound together to a lesser degree than in fibre, hence the body can completely digest starch, while it is not able to fully digest fibre. Starchy carbohydrates are nutrient rich (they contain fibre and micronutrients) but they are energy dense. If your portions of starchy carbs are consistently too large, your body can also convert the glucose in the starch into fat.

Starchy carbs include:

> root vegetables such as potatoes, beetroot and parsnips
> whole grains such as oats, wild rice, barley and quinoa
> products made from grains such as breads, crackers or breakfast cereals.

Fibrous carbs include:

> vegetables and whole fruit
> beans and lentils (these are fibrous but also contain some starchy carbohydrates, so they are referred to as fibrous starches).

FIBRE

Fibre is a type of carbohydrate and refers to the parts of plant-based foods (vegetables, fruit, nuts, seeds, whole grains and legumes) that are not broken down or used by the body. Instead, these non-digestible parts make their way through the gut and contribute to our health in different ways. They nourish our estrobolome (see page 27), helping to balance our hormones; they keep our appetite in check by keeping us feeling fuller for longer; and they help regulate blood-sugar control.

Fibre is classified as either soluble, which dissolves in water, or insoluble, which doesn't dissolve. To receive the greatest health benefit, you need to eat a wide variety of high-fibre foods. Current UK guidelines recommend we should aim for 30 grams of fibre every day, yet in the UK, only one in twenty of us is actually eating enough.

WHAT HAPPENS WHEN WE EAT CARBS?

Carbs are digested and eventually broken down into glucose, which is absorbed into your bloodstream and raises your blood-sugar levels. The more carbohydrates you eat, the higher your blood-sugar rises after that meal.

Our blood-sugar levels need to be kept within certain parameters for optimal wellbeing – having too much or too little puts stress on the body. To keep your blood-sugar levels in the healthy range, your pancreas releases the

hormone insulin. When the glucose level goes up, insulin goes up. If you eat lots of carbs at a meal, more glucose means more insulin.

Chronic high levels of blood glucose (excessive hyperglycaemia) causes inflammation. When your blood-glucose levels always peak or drop outside the optimal range, your endocrine (hormone) system is put on high alert and focuses all its attention on trying to stabilise your levels. This is okay if it happens occasionally. But when it happens often, this is when the problems can begin.

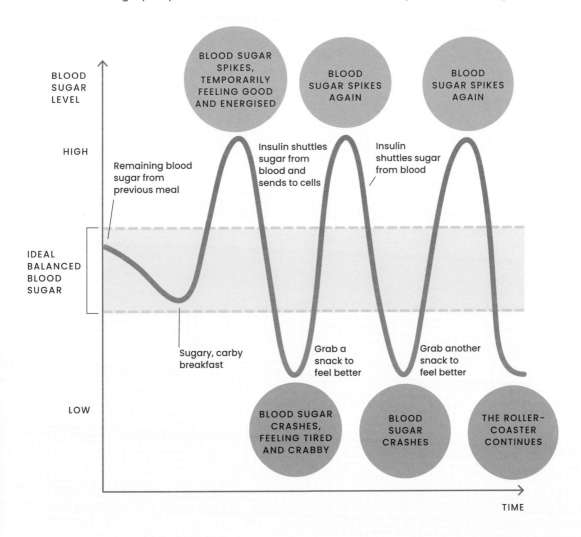

WHAT FOODS AFFECT YOUR BLOOD-SUGAR LEVELS?

The body handles various types of carbohydrates differently. Complex carbohydrates (whole grains, legumes, vegetables and whole fruit) that are rich in fibre are digested and absorbed slowly, which means a slow and gradual release of insulin.

In contrast, refined carbohydrates and sugar (white bread, sugary cereals, biscuits, cakes, white rice, sugar-laden drinks or even some 'healthy foods' that are very processed, like cereal bars or fruit yoghurt) are digested and absorbed rapidly, which means they cause a surge in blood-sugar levels and a consequent surge in insulin. The higher the rise, the more insulin you need. The more insulin you need, the quicker the drop in blood-sugar levels and the blood-sugar roller-coaster begins.

The glycaemic index

This index ranks foods numerically based on their effect on blood-sugar control. It shows how quickly individual foods containing carbohydrates affect your blood-sugar (glucose) levels, when eaten on their own. On this scale, glucose has the GI of 100. Other foods are ranked in relation to this. A GI of 55 or less is considered low, between 55–69 is medium, and above 70 is high. Several factors affect the GI of a food, such as what nutrients, other than carbs, are in the food, what you eat the carbs with, how the carbs are cooked, how much processing the food has gone through and how ripe the carb-rich food is. The riper or more mature the fruit is, the higher its GI.

Resist the urge to Google GI – you'll just get a long list of foods with numbers that may not mean that much. In general, there are some easy points to help you grasp the concept. Foods with a high GI are likely to be very processed. The more machines the food has been through, the higher the GI, as much of the 'digestion' has been done before consumption. For example, a cob of sweetcorn (lower GI) versus cornflakes (higher GI). Refined or ultra-processed foods have a high GI because they are rapidly digested and prompt swinging fluctuations in blood glucose. Conversely, unrefined carbs, whole foods, like whole oats, sweet potatoes, lentils and vegetables, have a low GI, because they are digested more slowly and prompt a more gradual rise in blood glucose.

As a rule, nutrition experts recommend you base your main meals on lower-GI carbs. However, while GI is a good guide when it comes to choosing carbohydrates, it shouldn't be used in isolation; you also need to consider the nutrient density of the food. Let's take a Mars bar versus a slice of watermelon as an example – a Mars bar has a GI of 56–69, which is considered moderate, while a slice of watermelon has a GI of 70–80, which is considered high. If you're just looking at GI, the chocolate bar appears to be healthier than the watermelon! Yet the watermelon contains more vitamins and minerals.

Whether you eat a food on its own or as part of a meal also matters. Mixing your carbs with some protein or fat is the way to go. This will reduce the speed at which the glucose is absorbed. For example, if you put some roast chicken (protein) and salad (low GI) on a white baguette (high GI), this brings down the overall GI of the bread.

Your portion sizes matter too. The 'glycaemic load' is a measure that helps you account for both the quantity and quality of your carbohydrates. This means that even if you eat a low-GI food like quinoa, if you eat the whole packet, your blood-sugar levels will go up, as it will be a larger carbohydrate load that your body has to deal with at one time.

We will talk more about portion control a little later but, as always with nutrition, the take-home message is moderation. When it comes to blood-sugar control, the type of carbohydrates you eat and the amount you eat both matter.

THE ROLLER-COASTER EFFECT AND YOUR HORMONES

It is commonly cited that there are 34 different menopause symptoms, and blood-sugar control is linked to almost all of them. Here are some of the main symptoms that are affected by fluctuating blood-sugar levels.

Your mood

Think about how you feel when your blood-sugar levels are low. (I know that low-blood-sugar Linia is not the nicest person; she is tired, irritable, moody and lightheaded, i.e. hangry!)

Every cell in your body depends on glucose for energy. For example, when your brain is low on glucose, it will not send or receive messages properly. This is why things like focus and memory are negatively impacted. Low blood-sugar levels may also make you feel anxious, worried, frustrated and panicked. Some people even get palpitations and headaches when their blood sugar drops.

Your weight

The bad news is that if you are on a blood-sugar roller-coaster, you are setting your body up to lose muscle tone and gain fat. Here's why.

Say you start the day with a refined-carbohydrate breakfast like toast, jam and a smoothie (mostly all carbs). Your blood-sugar levels will spike and you'll experience a temporary energy buzz, followed by a subsequent crash at mid-morning due to an overzealous surge of insulin that was needed to lower your high blood-sugar levels. Once your blood-sugar levels drop below the normal range, this puts your body on high alert. You will get a massive sugar craving. But if you can't get your hands on a tea or coffee and a KitKat, your body will produce adrenaline (one of the stress hormones). Adrenaline then breaks down some of your precious muscle to produce some glucose to push your blood-sugar levels up again.

Add to this the fact that chronically elevated blood-sugar levels increase your risk of putting on weight. Insulin's job is to help store nutrients, including fat. When there is an excess of glucose, insulin shunts glucose from your blood to your muscles and your liver to be stored for future energy needs. If these two storage spots are full, insulin sends the glucose to your fat cells, contributing to weight gain.

Hot flushes and fatigue

We are still learning about the link between hot flushes and blood sugar, although it seems clear that maintaining a stable blood-sugar level is sensible. Low blood sugars are thought to trigger hot flushes. In contrast, those who have worse hot flushes are at higher risk of diabetes,

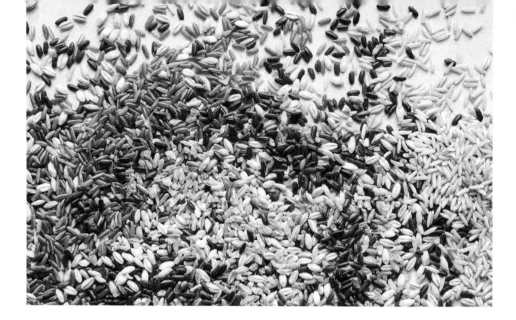

suggesting a link between higher sugars and worse symptoms.

Feeling tired is a common symptom in menopause and fluctuating blood-sugar levels can make you feel exhausted and lethargic.

Poor sleep quality

This is a bit of a chicken-and-egg scenario. Poor sleep causes you to crave sugar. However, too much sugar has been shown to disrupt the delicate balance of insulin, serotonin, dopamine and neurotransmitters, which can lead to sleep disturbances. It's thought that a high-sugar diet has a negative impact on sleep, particularly on the deepest and most restorative stage of the sleep cycle.

LONG-TERM EFFECTS

In the long term, elevated blood-glucose levels increase our risk of obesity, type 2 diabetes, dementia and heart disease. The mechanism for this is through something called insulin resistance. To explain this, I'll use a plant analogy. I love plants. I like to think I have green fingers but I don't. The reality is, I end up killing most of my plants as I over-water them. Plants need water to live, however if you over-water them, they die. We are much more complex than plants, however in a similar way, our endocrine systems depend on receiving the right kind of signals in the right amounts. Too much and it's overkill. Insulin resistance occurs when there is too much insulin circulating in your body and your cells stop listening to the insulin asking them to take glucose into their cells. As a result, insulin needs to shout louder to get the job done. This means more insulin is produced. Over time, this increases your risk of most chronic diseases.

NAILING YOUR CARBOHYDRATE INTAKE

Don't cut out carbs

The amount of carbs we should consume is a highly debated topic. Take weight loss, for example. Ask someone what they need to do to lose weight and one of the responses you will get will probably be: 'Cut back on the carbs'. Though limiting your carbs can lead to weight loss, eating carbs won't make you gain weight if you are eating the right ones in the right amounts. Although it is possible to survive on a very low-carb diet, it's probably not the optimal choice for the long term for most women in their menopause transition. Here's why:

> **The deprivation factor:** Perimenopause is not a time for deprivation. It's a time to learn to nourish your body. So, I want you to move away from the extreme idea of restricting and focus on adding quality nutrients. When done as a lifestyle change, this should become your new normal.

> **The gut health factor:** Study after study is showing how important maintaining a diversity of gut bacteria is for our waistline and health. To maintain this diversity, you need to include carbs in the form of whole grains, fruit and vegetables. They contain types of fibre that are known to have a 'prebiotic' effect. Prebiotics are nutrients that support the growth and activity of the healthy bacteria in your gut. Research shows that following a very low-carb diet for too long can negatively affect the diversity of our gut bacteria.

> **The sustainability factor:** Carb reduction costs us over the long term as we require some complex carbs to function at our best. Extreme diets almost never work as they are unsustainable. The key with carbohydrate intake is 'strategic moderation'. As unsexy as that sounds, it works and is sustainable.

WHO COULD BENEFIT FROM A LOW-CARB DIET?
Very sedentary people, as well as those who have insulin resistance (see opposite), may benefit from a lower-carb diet for a while as part of an overall transition towards more activity and a healthier metabolism.

I like 'treats' and 'junk food' as much as anyone else ... It comes back to one of my favourite words: balance.

Choose the right carbs

Not all carbs are created equal and here lies the challenge. The first thing I need to make clear is that we all need to keep our intake of simple carbs/free sugars to a minimum. The current guidelines are to reduce your sugar intake to less than 5 per cent of your total energy per day (30 grams per day or six teaspoons for adults), however, for most people, the less sugar the better.

As we know, refined sugars (biscuits, cakes, many breakfast cereals, overcooked pasta, sticky white rice and alcohol) are not good for blood-glucose levels as they create a blood-sugar roller-coaster. Foods with a low glycaemic index (such as whole grains, beans and lentils) release sugar into the blood more slowly. See the table below for smart swaps you can make.

Movement and carb intake

Movement influences your blood-glucose levels. Being more active improves your body's ability to use insulin to bring your blood-sugar levels down. That's why, after a carb-heavy meal, a gentle walk is a great idea. On sedentary days, researchers also recommend 'exercise snacks' to lower blood-sugar levels. Exercise snacking just means that you break up your sitting time every hour or so for a few minutes by doing some calf raises or squats or going for a light walk.

Simple carbs	Smart swap
Sugary breakfast cereal	Homemade muesli or granola or try my tasty Overnight oats on page 111
Instant oats	Porridge oats or try my Quinoa porridge on page 116
White bagels, bread or wraps	Wholegrain or seeded varieties or make your own!
Short-grain white rice	Brown, red and black rice, farro, quinoa
Cooked pasta	Al dente cooked pasta
Rice cakes	Oatcakes or dark rye crackers
Fruit juice	Whole fruit
Milk chocolate	Dark chocolate, at least 70 per cent cocoa solids

Get the portions right

One size doesn't fit all and this is true when it comes to portion sizes. There are different methods used to advise on portion sizes: plate guides, hand guides, weight guides and household measurement guides. No matter which guide you use, the key is to remember that they are just guides. People all have different needs and if you want tailored advice to suit your particular needs, seek support from a dietitian or nutritionist.

As a starting-off point, here is some portion advice using the plate guide. Divide your plate into sections based on different food groups. In general, for each meal I would recommend:

> vegetables, salad or lower-GI fruit: half a plate or two fistfuls
> protein: quarter of a plate
> complex carbs (such as whole grains, grains or starchy vegetables like potatoes and parsnips): quarter of a plate or one fistful.

Get the timing right

You've probably heard the saying: 'Eat breakfast like a king, lunch like a prince and dinner like a pauper', but how true is it really?

Our body's internal clock, known as the sleep-wake cycle, is controlled by our pituitary gland and it is what tells us we're sleepy. If you get enough sleep, you may notice you have slight dips in energy from 1–3pm (and if you're a shift worker, you'll have one again in the early morning from 2–4am).

Interestingly, some research also suggests that this is why our body is best primed to digest and metabolise food, particularly carbohydrates, at certain times of day. So, as a woman in your forties and above, I would recommend you have your starchy carbs at breakfast and lunch and then, based on your activity levels, rethink dinner and keep it low in starchy carbs.

I also tend to find this strategy works for most women as the evenings are our emotionally vulnerable times – we are tired. This means our willpower may be weakening. One small fistful of al dente pasta can turn into a big bowl with extra cheese added on top! If you are great with portion size and are super active, then, fantastic, you can have a fistful of carbs at dinner. If not, be mindful! This doesn't mean you have to cook another whole meal that's separate to the rest of the family's. You just need to cook more cleverly. I will help set you up for that in the recipe section.

Play the 80/20 game

Do I eat cake? Yes. Do I munch on crisps? Absolutely. I like 'treats' and 'junk food' as much as anyone else – whether that's a glass of wine, a bowl of chips or a slice of good cake.

The reality is there is no such thing as a 'bad' food; too much of anything can be bad. It comes back to one of my favourite words: balance. If you eat in balance most of the time (80 per cent), then some of your favourite treats, like cake or pizza, can be the remaining 20 per cent of your diet. That's also the most pleasurable way to eat, and it's why this book includes weekend indulgences. The key is to have these in moderation.

Note: if you want to drive fat loss and have some specific health goals, then the 80/20 game may need to become 95 per cent and 5 per cent for a period. The 80/20 game is for weight maintenance.

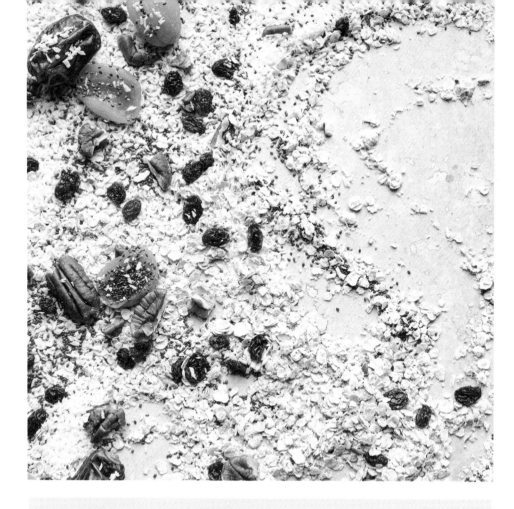

TAKEAWAYS

1. Managing blood-sugar levels is the cornerstone to good hormonal health. Excessive fluctuations lead to mood swings and low energy in the short term, a change of body shape in the medium term and an increased risk of chronic diseases, like type 2 diabetes, in the long term.

2. Opt for whole foods or high-fibre carbohydrates with a low GI that are slow to digest. Fibre slows the rate that the stomach empties, which has a knock-on effect on the rate of absorption of glucose in the bloodstream.

3. Don't eat your carbohydrates naked. Dress them. Meals without protein, fat or fibre are rapidly broken down and absorbed into the bloodstream.

4. In general, movement will lower your blood-sugar levels. Fuel appropriately for exercise to prevent dips in your blood sugar afterwards. After a big meal, a brisk walk can help rebalance blood-sugar regulation.

5. You are unique. One size doesn't fit all. For bespoke advice about your carbohydrate intake, it's recommended you see a registered dietitian or nutritionist.

WHAT IS PROTEIN?

Proteins are the building blocks of life and every living cell in the body uses them for both structural and functional purposes. Proteins are made from smaller molecules called amino acids, which link together, a little like Lego. The amino acids that are produced by your body are called non-essential amino acids; the ones you cannot produce are called essential amino acids, and you must get these from your diet.

Animal sources of protein tend to deliver all the amino acids we need to make new protein, but plant proteins don't. So, if you are vegetarian or vegan, it's important that your diet contains a wide variety of plant-based foods.

WHY IS PROTEIN SO IMPORTANT?

Protein ticks a lot of boxes and it's kinda a big deal for women, yet most women I see don't eat enough protein. It is particularly important for women aged forty and above due to its key role in the following functions.

Hormone production

Protein is needed to produce and transport hormones around the body. At a point in your life when hormone production is decreasing, it's vital to have sufficient building blocks for your key hormones.

Muscle growth and repair

As we age, we lose muscle mass naturally due to a process called sarcopenia. A 2021 study that compared women in early and late perimenopause found those in late perimenopause had 9 per cent lower muscle mass. Eating enough protein can help prevent muscle loss. The more muscle you have, the more calories your body burns at rest because muscles are more metabolically active than fat tissue. You are also more sensitive to insulin if you have more muscle. Less muscle means a lower capacity to store glucose, making it easier for your body to store carbs as fat.

Appetite regulation and blood-sugar control

When eaten with carbohydrates, protein slows the rate of carbohydrate absorption. Protein-rich foods also tend to make you feel fuller for longer. Distributing your protein intake throughout the day and including a lean protein source at each meal can help with appetite regulation and blood-sugar control.

Bone health

Physiologically, bones are not just walls of calcium – 50 per cent of your bone structure is protein. Following a low-protein diet weakens your bones.

Mood regulation

Your brain uses the amino acids found in protein to create key neurotransmitters that govern mood, memory and motivation – all of which can be problems for women in midlife.

Healthy aging

Protein is crucial to support healthy aging. Aging bodies process protein less efficiently and therefore you need more of it to maintain muscle mass and strength. The more muscle you have, the less frail you will be as you age.

As we age, our bodies begin to use protein less efficiently, so it's even more important that we eat enough of it.

WHICH FOODS CONTAIN PROTEIN?

It's not just about the quantity of the protein you eat; the quality matters too. Protein can come from animal or plant foods such as:

> meat, chicken and fish
> eggs
> nuts and seeds
> dried beans and lentils
> dairy products such as milk, yoghurt and cheese
> soy products.

It's important to eat a variety of protein foods. If you eat animal protein, choose lean sources such as chicken, turkey and fish (you should eat both white and oily fish). If you have red meat, enjoy it in moderation.

If you're a meat eater, be sure to serve up some vegetarian meals. Traditional plant-based proteins like beans, lentils and tofu are a great addition to the diet. Soy-based foods also contain isoflavones which may help to reduce hot flushes and night sweats in some women.

Processed meats

Processed meats, such as bacon, ham and sausages, should be eaten sparingly as they have been linked to an increased risk of cancer. Recommendations are that we have a maximum of 50 grams of processed meat per day. There are no guidelines on processed plant-based products (which include fake bacon, lab meat and veggie sausages or burgers), but I suggest that, as with processed meat, you keep your intake to a minimum.

When it comes to sausages, there are both good and not so good. In general,

read the label. Do you recognise the ingredients? What is the meat content? For meat sausages, the higher the meat percentage, the better. Buying them from a butcher is a good way of ensuring the quality, but if you can only buy from the supermarket, that's fine – just don't have them as often.

HOW MUCH PROTEIN SHOULD WE EAT?

As we age and go through the menopause transition, our bodies begin to use protein less efficiently, so it's even more important that we eat enough of it.

The 'right' amount of protein for an individual depends on many factors including age, level of activity, body composition, current state of health, goals and so on. In the UK, for adults, the reference nutrient intake (RNI) daily allowance is set at 0.75 grams of protein per kilogram of body weight per day. There are no specific protein guidelines for menopausal women, however a recent study from the European Society for Clinical and Economic Aspects of Osteoporosis, Osteoarthritis and Musculoskeletal Diseases (ESCEO) suggests that perimenopausal women should get a minimum of 1.2 grams of protein per kilogram of body weight per day.

The more active you are, the more protein you need. The extra protein helps with repair and rebuilds muscle cells that are damaged during exercise. Active women should be on 1.2–2.0 grams of protein per kilogram of body weight per day. This would mean a 70-kilogram woman should consume around 84–140 grams of protein per day. Remember, going above the recommendations isn't a smart move. It's about that B-word again – balance.

The best way to consume protein is to spread your intake across the day. Here's what 20 grams of protein can look like:

> 2 eggs and 2 slices of seeded toast
> 2 slices of wholemeal toast with 1 tablespoon peanut butter and a latte
> 125g Greek yoghurt with pumpkin seeds sprinkled on top
> 1 cup of cottage cheese with 1 apple
> Small chicken breast or ½ a big chicken breast
> 75g smoked or poached salmon
> 1 cup of cooked edamame or cooked lentils.

TIP: A palm-size serving of animal protein (chicken, fish or meat) is about 30 grams of protein. Protein should be a quarter of your plate.

WHAT ABOUT PROTEIN POWDERS?

The answer is always: food first, because whole foods come packaged with other nutrients like vitamins, minerals and phytochemicals. No supplement will be able to imitate the exact combinations, nor their synergistic effects. But if you want the convenience of a protein powder, here are my tips for choosing a good one.

> Choose a protein powder with as few additives as possible. Unflavoured powders are a good starting point.
> If you have a flavoured protein powder with sweeteners, for optimal gut health, use it a couple of times a week rather than daily.
> Choose a brand that has had third-party testing where possible. Look for certifications from organisations such as Informed Sport, Informed Choice, USP and NSF.

TAKEAWAYS

1. Women in their forties and over need to prioritise their protein intake. Not only is it integral to hormonal production, it also helps reduce muscle loss, supports appetite regulation and blood-sugar control and helps with mood regulation.

2. Eat enough protein at the right times. The more active you are, the more protein you need. It's important to spread your protein intake out throughout the day.

3. Quality matters. Keep it lean. Reduce your intake of processed protein from both animal and plant sources.

4. Include some meat-free meals in your menu. Plant-based proteins like beans and lentils are great for winter soups and stews.

5. Food first. Try to get your protein from whole food. If you want to use a protein powder, choose one that has had as little added to it as possible.

FATS

Fat is bad. No, fat is good. Actually … some fats are better than others. It's confusing, isn't it?

To understand fat, you need to know there are different types of fats with different chemistries, which affect their health benefits. All fats have a similar overall structure: a chain of carbon atoms bonded to hydrogen atoms. What makes one fat different from another is the length and shape of the carbon chain and the number of hydrogen atoms. Depending on their chemical structure, fats are classified as saturated or unsaturated.

Types of fats

Saturated fats consist of a straight chain of carbon atoms. This flat structure allows them to stack easily, forming solids at room temperature. Examples of saturated fats include butter, lard and coconut oil.

The healthier fats are called unsaturated fats. Of these, monounsaturated fats have a kink in the carbon chain, making them less prone to congregate and allowing them to stay liquid at room temperature. Examples include olive oil and avocado oil. Polyunsaturated fats are also called 'essential' fats, meaning we need to include them in our diet. Structurally, they have more kinks, allowing them to stay liquid at cold temperatures. A good example is fish oil. Within the polyunsaturated fat family, you get omega-3 fats and omega-6 fats.

Ideally, we need to have a balance of both omega-3 and 6. Unfortunately, in our modern Western diets, we are not eating enough anti-inflammatory omega-3 and eating too many refined sources of omega-6 (i.e. refined sunflower and soybean oil or deep-fried food).

THE GOOD	THE 'BAD'	THE UGLY
Unsaturated fats	Saturated fats	Trans fats
Can be eaten regularly. Watch the portion size.	Should be eaten less often. Watch the portion size.	Limit.
Avocado Olives and olive oil Cold-pressed rapeseed oil Nuts and seeds Oily fish	Butter Dairy products Red meat Cheese Lard Goose fat Coconut oil Coconut cream Ghee	Hardened margarine Fried fast food Some packaged baked goods or snack foods

Trans fats are a byproduct of a process called hydrogenation. Hydrogenation is used by the food industry to turn liquid vegetable oils into solid fats, therefore giving them more desirable physical properties (i.e. longer shelf life). Trans fats increase the risk of heart attacks, strokes and type 2 diabetes.

Foods tend to contain a mix of both unsaturated and saturated fats, however they tend to be classed within whichever type is highest.

WHY GOOD FATS ARE IMPORTANT DURING THE MENOPAUSE

Fat is not the enemy and menopause is not a time for following a zero-fat or super-low-fat diet. Including healthy fats in your diet is crucial for the following reasons.

Hormone production

We need a certain amount of fat in our diet to produce hormones, including our sex hormones. The menopause is the point in your life where you need all the hormones you can get!

Brain health

The human brain is 60 per cent fat, so following a super-low-fat diet during the menopause will only make brain fog and forgetfulness worse.

Absorption of essential vitamins

Vitamins A, D, E and K are fat soluble, meaning they need fat in order to be absorbed and used properly in the body. Vitamin A is needed for healthy skin and the immune system. Vitamin D is not just needed for your bones; it's needed pretty much everywhere. Vitamin E is another skin essential but also supports a healthy heart.

Vitamin K is an unsung bone-health hero.

Weight management

Believe it or not, including healthy fats in your diet will help you control your cravings and your weight. Which is more satisfying, salmon or cod? Most people would say salmon. That's because it has a higher proportion of healthy fats and fats are satiating – they fill you up and satisfy you, so you are more likely to eat less.

Skin health

Every cell in your body has a little layer of fat in it. Fat is important for general cellular health – and the skin is no exception. Our skin changes during the menopause due to the decline in oestrogen, so having healthy fats in your diet can keep your skin glowing.

Joint support

Joint pain and inflammation are common symptoms in the menopause (my knees sound like they need oiling most of the time!). Good fats provide the building blocks that make up the lubrication our joints need. Some fats are also anti-inflammatory, but I'll go into that in more detail later.

LESS IS MORE

I haven't talked a lot about calories. I'm not a fan of hard-core calorie counting as it's a simplified and not very meaningful bit of nutrition science. However, although we don't need to obsess about calorie counting, calories do count, and fats are calorific compared to other foods. To give you some perspective, 1 gram of protein and 1 gram of carbohydrates is 4.2 calories, 1 gram of alcohol is 7.5 calories, and 1 gram of fat is 9 calories.

Just because avocado is good for you, it doesn't mean eating two a day is a good idea!

Fat is energy dense, so you need to make sure you get your portion sizes right. Just because avocado is good for you, it doesn't mean eating two a day is a good idea! Two avocados would be about 500 calories, which is a quarter of the recommended average daily calorie intake for women.

Don't assume that fat-free is healthier, either. Many fat-free products have added sugar (to make the products taste better), so have a look at the ingredient list.

HOW MUCH FAT?

The advice differs, but in the UK, the Dietary Reference Intake (DRI) for adults says you should get 20–30 per cent of your total daily calories from fat. Since the recommended average female calorie allowance per day is 2000 calories, this would equate to approximately 45–75 grams per day. Within this, we are advised that our saturated fat intake should not exceed 11 per cent of the total energy from food, which is roughly 20 grams per day for women. Trans fats should be kept to a minimum, however the guidelines are that they should be no more than 2 per cent of our daily intake.

We need to be increasing our intake of essential fatty acids, especially omega-3s. It's recommended that we eat two portions of fish per week, one of which should be oily fish (one portion is 140 grams fresh fish or one small can). Plant-based omega-3 sources include walnuts, flaxseeds, pumpkin seeds and seaweed.

In practice, this means that at every meal, you can have one to two fat portions based on your activity levels.

One portion is approximately:

> 1 tablespoon extra virgin olive oil
> Half an avocado
> 30 grams seeds or nuts
> 1 tablespoon nut butter
> 30 grams cheese (the size of a standard matchbox)
> 8 olives
> 5 grams butter, about 1 teaspoon.

HEALTHY FATS

Superfoods don't exist. However, there are some healthy fats that are good for you to regularly add to your diet, particularly in your menopause years (they are included in the recipes too).

1. **Extra virgin olive oil.** It's rich in heart-healthy monounsaturated fats and a compound called oleocanthal, which has anti-inflammatory properties. It's a key part of the Mediterranean diet.

2. **Nuts.** Nuts are nutrient-packed powerhouses. They give you protein, healthy fats and antioxidants, all vital for healthy hormones. Go for unsalted, unroasted varieties. Try to eat a variety of different nuts – and don't eat the whole bag! Keep it to a handful.

3. **Seeds.** Pumpkin seeds, flaxseeds, chia seeds, sunflower and sesame seeds are some of the best multi-tasking foods around. They are high in fibre and contain antioxidants which help fight free radicals in the body. They are also high in omega-3, known as alpha-linolenic acid (ALA), which supports skin health, and are rich in minerals. I'm a big fan of a seed mix.

4. **Dark chocolate.** Dark chocolate contains flavanols that act as antioxidants in the body. Research

suggests that flavanols slow down damage caused by free radicals and have powerful anti-inflammatory properties, which may improve skin health and help you age better. But the research also shows that there needs to be at least 70 per cent cocoa content for there to be any real benefit. A portion is 20–30 grams (two to three squares), not the whole bar.

5. Oily fish. Salmon, sardines, trout, mackerel and mussels are high in omega-3s, protein, selenium and an antioxidant called astaxanthin, which are all associated with maintaining strong muscles and healthy bones, and reducing inflammation.

6. Eggs. These are 'egg-cellent' (sorry! I couldn't resist) sources of protein, but they provide some fats and key vitamins and minerals as well. Eggs also contain lecithin, which is a source of a nutrient called choline. Research shows that diets rich in choline can lead to a sharper memory. Keep your intake of eggs to six to eight a week.

7. Bio-live Greek yoghurt. Greek yoghurt is a multitasker too. It's high in protein, contains live bacteria that support gut health and is a great source of calcium. I opt for full-fat as I like the creaminess; I just have a smaller portion. If you opt for low-fat, check the label to ensure it contains only milk and live bacteria cultures.

8. Avocado. From toast toppings to salads and desserts, this versatile food is high in healthy fats and a good source of vitamin E, folate and fibre.

TAKEAWAYS

1. Get over your fat phobia! We need to include some fat in our diet, especially during the menopause, for hormone production, brain health, absorption of essential vitamins and minerals, weight management and skin health.

2. Include essential fatty acids in your diet – have a handful of raw nuts and seeds a day, and eat oily fish, such as mackerel, salmon, fresh tuna or sardines, at least once a week.

3. All researchers still agree that trans fats are the worst – try to avoid these as much as possible. Look out for 'partially hydrogenated' or 'hydrogenated' on food labels.

4. Keep on top of your fat portion sizes. Don't forget that all types of fat are still very calorie dense and, as with all foods, overeating will lead to weight gain if the calories you eat exceed the calories you burn.

5. Ensure you're getting the right amount of fat for your individual needs. Getting advice from a dietitian or nutritionist is a good place to start.

What a balanced plate looks like

Let's bring it all together now. We know that balanced blood-sugar levels have far-reaching effects on your menopausal symptoms and your wellbeing in the short and long term. Keeping your blood-sugar levels in check means serving up a balanced plate.

1. Always start by adding lots of veggies and some fruit. The more colour, the better.

2. Prioritise protein and add it next. Keep it lean.

3. Add in the wholegrain carbs based on your activity levels, personal goals and time of day.

4. Top it all off with some healthy fat. Be portion wise.

5. Add some other plants like herbs and spices.

WHAT ABOUT SNACKS?

There has been much research into snacking in an attempt to establish what impact it has on nutrition and health outcomes, but there is no clear answer. Whether snacks affect appetite and weight seems to depend on the individual, the type of snack consumed and the timing of the snack. My take? Snacking is fine as long as you snack smart!

Reflect on a typical day. When are you snacking? Midmorning? Midafternoon? Before dinner is cooked? If you're snacking often, try to work out why. If you find yourself snacking because you're bored, stressed or tired, start checking in with your emotions more regularly and look for other ways to meet your emotional needs.

Snack smart

A snack portion should be enough to satisfy but not so much that it interferes with your appetite or adds too many calories. In general, it's best to eat snacks that provide about 200 calories and at least 5–10 grams of protein to help you stay full until your next meal.

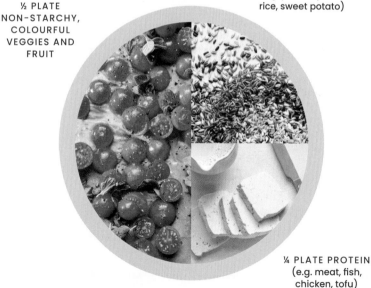

½ PLATE NON-STARCHY, COLOURFUL VEGGIES AND FRUIT

¼ PLATE STARCHY CARBOHYDRATE (e.g. potato, pasta, rice, sweet potato)

¼ PLATE PROTEIN (e.g. meat, fish, chicken, tofu)

Try to snack on whole foods that contain a combination of nutrients. A combination of protein, fibre, whole grains and some 'good fats' is best (such as a piece of fruit and a closed handful of nuts, or some raw carrots with 2 tablespoons of hummus, or a handful of my Crispy roast chickpeas on page 154).

CAN I EAT FRUIT?

Yes, you can and you should! When you consume whole fruit, the natural sugars are bound within the structure (intrinsic sugar), so they hit your bloodstream more slowly than when you consume sugary food and drinks. Juicing loses the fibre in the whole fruit and releases the sugar from the cell's walls (extrinsic sugars); this is why fruit juice contains free sugars. Therefore, the recommendations are that we limit our intake of fruit juice and shop-bought smoothies to 150 millilitres per day. The good news is that homemade smoothies can count as two portions, depending on the amount of pulp (fibre) they contain. Blending is when the whole fruit or vegetable is used; what you put into the blender is what you consume.

WHAT'S THE DEAL WITH GLUTEN?

Gluten is a protein found in wheat, barley, rye, spelt and, to a lesser extent, oats. Originally, gluten-free diets were designed to combat coeliac disease, which is an autoimmune disorder characterised by a permanent intolerance to gluten. Gluten intolerance or sensitivity is a term used to describe individuals who can't tolerate gluten (they experience symptoms such as gas, bloating and lethargy) but who don't have coeliac disease. During the menopause, hormonal changes can affect the gut, and may mean that women suffer more with food intolerances, including to gluten.

From my clinical experience, I have found that it comes down to the individual as we all react differently. Keep in mind the following:

1. If you think you have coeliac disease, see your doctor. Losing weight, being deficient in iron (anaemic) or having a family history of coeliac disease are all good prompts to talk to a doctor.

2. Keep a food and symptom diary. Signs of gluten intolerance to look out for after eating gluten-rich foods include bloating, cramping, constipation, diarrhoea and fatigue.

3. If you think you may be sensitive to gluten, you could trial a couple of weeks without eating gluten and see how you feel. You'll need to get good at reading labels as gluten is very often found in places you wouldn't expect, like supplements, salad dressings or veggie burgers.

4. Not all grains contain gluten. You've got lots of options, including quinoa, buckwheat, amaranth, millet and rice.

5. Remember, just because it's gluten free doesn't necessarily mean it's healthier. Many gluten-free products are filled with sugar, additives and preservatives that are not good for you if eaten too regularly either.

6. Before cutting out gluten completely, see a dietitian or registered nutritionist. They'll assist you with an elimination diet and help you ascertain your level of tolerance.

Principle 3: Feeding your gut bacteria

We women are pretty awesome for many reasons, but one of our super powers is our intuition, or our 'gut feelings'. It turns out there is really something to this. The gut has a direct impact on our internal state and wellbeing, and is often called the 'second brain'. It literally runs the show in your body.

YOUR MAGIC MICROBIOME

As explained on page 26, the gut is home to trillions of microorganisms that are collectively referred to as the microbiome. As well as digesting food, the microbiome helps to regulate your metabolism, your hormones and your mood, and it influences your immune system and your risk of disease. Science in this area is still evolving, and we are discovering more each day about the importance of good gut health. Below is an overview of some of the ways that your microbiome impacts your health, and why women in their forties and over particularly need to prioritise their gut health.

Hormone balance

The gut microbiome is one of the main regulators of circulating oestrogen, via the estrobolome (see page 27 for more on how this works). Bacteria in your estrobolome are also little manufacturing centres – they can make oestrogen from plants in our diet. They do this by converting compounds called phytoestrogens (found in soy-based foods) and lignans (found in legumes, whole grains and flaxseeds). Phytoestrogens are incredibly important because when your oestrogen levels are high, they can block the receptors and protect you from the risks of excess oestrogen exposure, and when oestrogen is low they can provide enough to keep your levels supported.

Your weight

Your gut bacteria and other microorganisms in your gut help you digest food, absorb nutrients and also determine where you store energy. They are mostly composed of two dominant bacterial groups, one of which absorbs more energy than the other. If your gut flora is out of balance, some research suggests that you can begin to extract more calories (i.e. energy) from your food, experience more cravings and feel hungry all the time, which makes managing your weight more difficult.

Your brain

Many of your neurotransmitters, the brain's chemical messengers, are controlled and produced by the bacteria in your gut. Serotonin, the mood regulator and happy hormone, is a major one. Roughly 95 per cent of your body's serotonin is produced in the gut. There are many connections between the gut and the brain. The gut–brain axis is the highway of connection between the intestine and the emotional and cognitive centres of the brain. There is a lot about brain health we still don't know, but we do know the microbiome is a vital part of the puzzle.

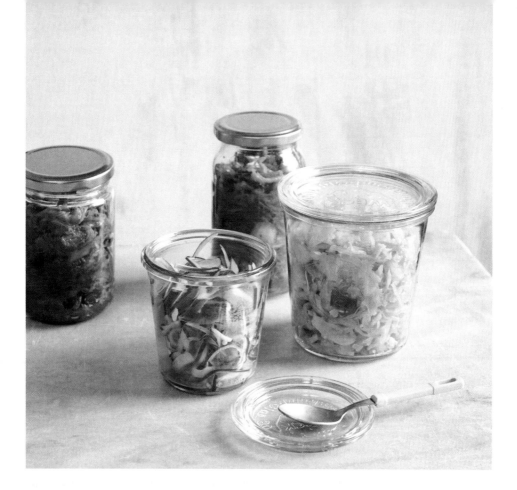

Sleep

Studies show that the gut microbiome can influence sleep quality. Good sleep depends on many different factors but what is interesting is that one study found that having a more diverse microbiome was linked with better sleep.

Inflammation and disease

A healthy microbiome supports a healthy immune system. Many factors, especially antibiotics, smoking, stress and a diet high in refined carbs, can disrupt the microbiome. This in turn can trigger an abnormal immune response and inflammation in the gut. But what happens in the gut does not stay in the gut. An inflamed gut can have far-reaching effects throughout the body.

At the current life expectancy, women will on average spend approximately one-third of their lives in postmenopause, which comes with an elevated risk of age-related chronic diseases that are possibly accelerated by the menopause transition. The bacterial mix in your microbiome can also influence the production of inflammatory chemicals, which overall creates an inflammatory environment in your body. It is now well established that low-grade, chronic inflammation is a common feature of pretty much all metabolic, psychiatric and neurodegenerative diseases.

Research suggests it can take as little as five days to change your microbiome for the better by eating the right kinds of foods.

WHAT IS A HEALTHY GUT?

Although no two microbiomes are identical, there are a few species of bacteria that are particularly common and make up a 'core' set of gut microbes for us all. There are five main families of bacteria. About two-thirds belong to a family called firmicutes and these contain lactobacilli, which have become the main bacteria used in probiotic supplements. The four other families contain bacteria such as bifidobacteria, clostridia, enterobacteriaceae, escherichia coli, and bacteroides to name a few (as well as thousands of bacteria that do not have a name yet).

Each of these different bacteria have distinct metabolisms and produce specific chemicals and hormones that interact with our gut and body in different ways. Your gut lining is also home to a network of approximately one hundred million neurons that are embedded in it, and the bacteria use this network to communicate among themselves and with the rest of your body.

Simply put, a healthy microbiome is made up of both 'good' and 'bad' bacteria, in specific amounts and located in specific places, that work together to create a harmonious ecosystem. If you remember the story of Goldilocks and the Three Bears, Goldilocks tried each porridge until she found the one that was 'just right'. It's kinda like that. If there is a disturbance in that balance – brought on by the prolonged use of antibiotics, or other bacteria-destroying medication, or a poor diet and unhealthy lifestyle – dysbiosis may occur. Dysbiosis is an imbalance in good and bad bacteria that can have a knock-on effect on gut health and often affects the permeability of your gut lining.

Two main states of dysbiosis exist. The first is a bacterial overgrowth, when certain bacterial species that you don't want in high levels get the upper hand and start to proliferate, disrupting the ecosystem. Or sometimes they end up in the wrong place (i.e. the small intestine). When any bacterial overgrowth occurs in your estrobolome (the part of your gut that metabolises oestrogen), this can elevate circulating oestrogen levels and lead to all sorts of hormone problems such as heavy periods, painful cramps, recurrent vaginal infections and mood swings. If this dysbiosis becomes chronic, it can increase your risk of endometriosis, fertility challenges, uterine fibroids and even breast and endometrial cancers.

On the flip side, dysbiosis can also occur if there aren't enough of the right types of microbes in your gut to metabolise oestrogens. The scientific term for this is 'low microbial diversity'. The consequences of this are twofold: first, your estrobolome can't adequately convert oestrogen to its active form and second, it also can't convert and use those protective plant-based oestrogens. This leads to low oestrogen overall.

WHAT HAPPENS TO THE GUT DURING MENOPAUSE?

The research on menopause and the gut microbiome has just begun. While some small human studies exist, we need a lot more quality research to really understand the relationship. Here's what we know so far.

1. Our gut microbiome changes over a lifetime, with the largest shift happening in early life during weaning,

when the diversity of the gut microbiome skyrockets from the transition from breast milk or substitute milk to solid food. In general, women are thought to have a more diverse microbiome than men. It's an X chromosome thing. Gut microbiome diversity appears to plateau around the age of forty.

2. There is a strong relationship between our sex hormones and gut microbiomes, and each influences the other. Higher levels of oestrogen and progesterone promote increased microbial diversity, which means you are healthier and have less severe menopausal symptoms.

3. During the menopause, as hormone levels decrease, if you're not on top of your gut game, the gut microbiome can become less diverse (some studies suggest that our gut microbiome starts looking more like a man's). Lower levels of oestrogen and progesterone also means your gut becomes more permeable, allowing 'microbial translocation', the movement of bacteria and their metabolites into areas where they wouldn't normally be.

4. Menopausal influence on the gut microbiome has broad consequences: mood swings, less restful sleep, more hot flushes, food cravings, low libido, inflammation, higher risk of diabetes, heart disease and dementia.

The good news (at last!) is you can do something about all this. The gut microbiome is modifiable. In fact, research suggests it can take as little as five days to change your microbiome for the better by eating the right kinds of foods. Ka-ching!

BALANCING YOUR ESTROBOLOME

By now the burning question you'll have is: how do I balance my estrobolome? How do I eat to help my gut bacteria during menopause when hormone levels are decreasing?

Studies show that the classic Western-style diet or the Standard American Diet (ironically SAD) has a negative effect on the microbiome. The SAD is devoid of fibre and antioxidants and is high in added sugar, refined carbs and ultra-processed foods. It also includes excessive amounts of meat and processed fats. These are all foods that, if eaten in excess, play havoc with the balance of bacteria in your gut, so we need to look at minimising them. Here's a rundown of how they can cause harm.

Sugar

Diets high in added sugar alter the microbiome by favouring the growth of unwanted species of bacteria that contribute to chronic inflammation, weight struggles and, over time, a 'leaky' gut.

Artificial sweeteners

Recent research has shown that our guts don't like large amounts of artificial sweeteners. Although diet versions of sweet products may help you reduce your calorie intake, based on evidence from animal studies, they may destroy the diversity of your gut microbiome if consumed habitually. We still don't know if some artificial sweeteners are better or worse than others. The message is that the occasional artificially sweetened drink is okay, but a habitual intake is not advisable. Whether you are better off having sugar instead of sweeteners will depend on a number of factors such as your medical history, your weight and your goals.

Ultra-processed foods

The exact definition of an ultra-processed food is up for debate, but in my clinical practice I tend to say that if the label has a super-long list of ingredients that you won't find in your kitchen, it's likely to be an ultra-processed food. Foods that are very high in added sugar, salt and fat are also likely to be ultra-processed. Examples include crisps, sugary breakfast cereals, biscuits, fizzy drinks, fruit-flavoured yoghurt and ice cream. A number of different theories on why ultra-processed foods are not good for us have been proposed, including that they are highly moreish, and the additives in them may negatively disrupt your gut health.

Alcohol

Alcohol inflames the gut and disrupts your microbiome. Interestingly, research also shows that alcohol can raise oestrogen levels in the short and long term and one of the ways it is thought to do this is by negatively impacting the estrobolome. This doesn't mean you have to become teetotal, however if you are struggling with your gut or your hormones, alcohol is a big one to watch. More on this later.

HEALTHY GUT, HEALTHY HORMONES

'You are what you eat' is a common saying. Given that our gut bacteria are so intricately linked with how well our entire body works, technically the saying should be: you are what your gut bacteria eat! Here are my top three ways that you can eat for a healthy gut, which will in turn ensure that your hormones are functioning at their best.

1. Make friends with fibre: Fibre feeds good bacteria – it's their absolute favourite food, and it tends to be one nutrient we don't eat enough of. 'Good' bacteria ferment the fibre in the large bowel, producing beneficial metabolites such as short-chain fatty acids that help to support a healthy digestive tract. They are also great sources of vitamins, minerals and other phytochemicals that promote health.

Eating more fibre will not only benefit your gut, it will have a positive impact on your waistline, your heart and pretty much every organ in your body.

2. Make it your mission to have a varied diet: Are you a routine kinda person when it comes to food? If it's a yes, then the chances are the diversity of your diet is low. Our gut bacteria love variety. American researchers found that people who ate about thirty different plant-based foods a week had a more diverse microbiome than those who were eating half that.

The colourful compounds (or polyphenols) found in a wide variety of plants serve as prebiotics, which our guts love. So eating the widest possible range of plant-based foods is a great way to maintain gut health.

One way to make this easier is by eating seasonally. In the UK, you can buy strawberries or asparagus any time of year. Yet, when I did my PhD in Milan, it was a travesty if I pulled out some grapes to snack on in January! Eating in season means the food is harvested and ripened at the right time and contains a greater amount of beneficial plant compounds.

3. Include fermented foods: The

process of fermenting involves bacteria and yeast, so it makes sense that increasing your intake of fermented foods has a positive impact on your gut microbiome. Some studies have linked the intake of fermented foods to better gut health and a reduced risk of cardiovascular disease and type 2 diabetes.

Kefir is the fermented food that has the most research behind it. It contains around twenty different types of bacteria and yeast. However, there are a range of foods, such as bio-live yoghurt, kimchi, sauerkraut, miso, tempeh, sourdough bread and even some mature cheeses, that are also believed to benefit the gut. Some fermented foods contain a lot of added sugar, though. Opt for plain varieties and look for the words 'live cultures'.

PLANT POINTS

Research has found that people who eat at least thirty different plant-based foods a week have a more diverse gut microbiome. Try this challenge to see how close you get. Even if you don't reach thirty, you'll do your gut a favour by adding more variety to your diet. Aim for four or five 'plant points' a day. Each plant counts as one point, while herbs and spices, extra virgin olive oil, tea and coffee count as quarter points.

- *Plant points are given for each variety of plant. So, if you eat two oranges, it only counts as one point!*
- *Fresh, frozen, canned or dried plant foods all count – however, be sure to aim for no-added-sugar and no-added-salt options.*
- *Only whole foods count. Refined or very processed plants such as white grains don't count. Fruit and vegetable juices also don't count.*

TAKEAWAYS

1. Eating to nourish your gut bacteria is paramount during the menopause as your hormones decrease your gut microbiome diversity and this can have a negative impact on all your symptoms and your long-term health.

2. What you eat can profoundly affect the balance of your 'good' and 'bad' bacteria. Reduce your intake of added sugar, artificial sweeteners and ultra-processed foods, and keep your alcohol intake low.

3. Fibre is a key player in achieving 'good' gut health, as it can be broken down by the bacteria in the microbiome, in turn providing fuel for their growth and activity.

4. Focus on variety. Eating a wide range of plant-based foods will lead to a more diverse gut microbiome. Aim for thirty different plant-based foods per week.

5. Include something fermented every day. Fermented foods like bio-live yoghurt, kefir, sauerkraut, kimchi and miso are packed with probiotics and eating them is one way to boost your gut health.

Principle 4: Eating to reduce inflammation

No battle is ever won or lost over a single meal; what's important is your overall eating pattern.

Each phase of the menopause comes with changes. These occur naturally because of the aging process, however they seem to be amplified by fluctuating hormone levels.

One of these changes is heightened activity of something called 'oxidative stress', when there is a mismatch between harmful free radicals and our body's capacity to neutralise them. Another change is our cellular powerhouses that generate energy (the mitochondria) become less efficient. This is why, at fifty, you don't typically run around with the energy of a five-year-old.

Another important change is a slow yet progressive increase in inflammation, known as chronic low-grade inflammation. We don't just see it happening on a cellular level. One recent study found women in the menopause appear to have more systemic inflammation. The relationship between menopause and inflammation is not fully understood, but we know it's an issue during and after the menopause. It can make symptoms worse and increases our risk of diseases like type 2 diabetes, heart disease, arthritis and dementia. Cooling inflammation is essential to a healthy menopause transition.

UNDERSTANDING INFLAMMATION

Inflammation happens in everyone, and it's not always a bad thing. There are two types: acute and chronic. Most people are familiar with acute inflammation: the redness, heat and swelling around tissues and joints when you cut your finger or bang your knee. When the body signals an injury or virus, your immune system sends out an army of white blood cells to surround and protect the area.

Chronic inflammation is a long-term physiological response that can last anywhere from weeks to years. Unlike acute inflammation, it's not visible to the naked eye. The same reaction takes place – white blood cells flood the problem area – but the 'flame' persists and the inflammation spreads through the body, creating destructive reactions that damage cells.

THE MENOPAUSE– INFLAMMATION LINK

Progesterone helps regulate inflammation in our body and brain. It also supports a healthy immune system, which is a key part of keeping inflammation at bay. Oestrogen is also anti-inflammatory and is thought to have an important role in regulating a key component of the innate immune responses (the inflammasome). During menopause, women with decreasing levels of oestrogen lose these anti-inflammatory effects, which results in the inflammasome part of the immune system becoming overactivated. This creates chronic low-grade inflammation. Decreasing levels of oestrogen also mean the brain is more susceptible to inflammation and neurodegenerative diseases, which may be one reason why women are more prone to dementia. However, there is still a lot we don't understand.

Increased weight gain, particularly around the waist (visceral fat), also affects inflammation. Visceral fat cells do more than store excess energy; they produce hormones and inflammatory substances.

WHAT ELSE CAUSES INFLAMMATION?

A poor diet

A diet high in the following foods is linked with an increase in inflammation:

> refined ultra-processed carbohydrates
> ultra-processed foods (junk food)
> high-fructose corn syrup
> trans fats
> processed meats
> alcohol.

It's important to note that no battle is ever won or lost over a single meal; what's important is your overall eating pattern.

Other lifestyle factors

Not getting enough sleep promotes inflammation. A recent study found people who sleep less than six hours per night or have disrupted sleep have higher levels of C-reactive protein, an acute marker of inflammation.

Research also shows long periods of sitting down, even for people who are active, can take a toll on your health. Sitting decreases circulation, encourages the body to shut down metabolically and increases the levels of inflammatory markers in your body.

Pollution can take its toll too. The World Health Organization (WHO) provides evidence of the links between long-term exposure to air pollution and type 2 diabetes, obesity and systemic inflammation. Managing stress is also important as it can cause inflammation. We talk more about this in part 3.

SYMPTOMS LINKED WITH INFLAMMATION

It's hard to pinpoint the symptoms that are linked to inflammation as it compromises your body's hormone production and muddles hormone signals everywhere. It makes us more susceptible to symptoms in general. Here are some you may end up feeling.

Pain

Oestrogen helps to lubricate joints and keep inflammation at bay. Higher levels of inflammation can cause achy joints. The relationship between menopause and increased pain is not well understood but we do know that oestrogens have complex interactions with pain-sensitivity receptors. Inflammation can make this worse.

Low mood and depression

A new study found high levels of a specific inflammatory molecule were associated with a higher likelihood of depressive symptoms, even after taking other factors, such as antidepressant use, into consideration.

DIETARY MANAGEMENT

Our daily food choices can be powerful tools to manage inflammation. There are foods that fan the flames of inflammation and those that cool. It isn't about a list of 'forbidden foods'. It's about making changes so the overall pattern is anti-inflammatory.

An anti-inflammatory eating pattern is based on whole foods, lots of vegetables and fruit and a balance of protein, wholegrain carbs and healthy fats at each meal.

TOP ANTI-INFLAMMATORY FOODS

The following foods have an anti-inflammatory link, however there is no magic bullet. Remember, it's about the context of your overall diet and lifestyle. You should include these foods regularly on your shopping list but mix them up. Variety is the spice of life. Including these 'hero' ingredients is fantastic, but please don't lose sight of the idea of balance and that everything works together.

1. Herbs and spices: All herbs and spices have some degree of antioxidant power, protecting us against oxidative stress. Turmeric, for example, has become renowned for its anti-inflammatory properties. Several trials suggest that curcumin (the active ingredient in turmeric) has beneficial effects on a range of inflammatory diseases. However, it's not easily absorbed by the body, meaning you must eat a lot of turmeric (at least seven teaspoons a day) for it to have any impact. Research also suggests garlic, ginger, rosemary, thyme and cinnamon all contain compounds that have potential anti-inflammatory effects.

2. Beans, lentils and whole grains: Keeping inflammation at bay means keeping your blood-sugar curve moderate. Focus on including whole grains, lentils and beans in your diet as your top carbohydrate choices, as they are fibre rich and are digested and absorbed slowly.

3. Green tea: Green tea contains a powerful antioxidant that has anti-inflammatory properties and is also thought to support the body to detoxify more effectively. Other good teas to include are ginger, rosehip, fennel and holy basil.

4. Omega-3-rich foods: Omega-3 fats are natural inflammation busters. They help to curb the production of inflammation-triggering molecules. Top sources include oily fish, walnuts, flaxseeds, pumpkin seeds and seaweed.

5. Fermented foods: Around 70–80 per cent of the immune cells are present in the gut, which is why optimising gut health is integral to promoting good immune health and eliminating chronic inflammation. Good gut health depends on having the right balance of bacteria and feeding them the right foods. Including one fermented food a day in your diet is a great way to keep your gut healthy.

6. Extra virgin olive oil (EVOO): EVOO has been studied for its protective benefits against inflammation. Olive oil's main anti-inflammatory effects are from antioxidants, one of which is called oleocanthal. It's thought to work like an anti-inflammatory drug.

7. Berries: From raspberries to blackberries, strawberries and blueberries, berries possess an abundance of bio-active compounds, such as anthocyanins and ellagic acid, that are anti-inflammatory. They are also rich in vitamin C, which is an antioxidant.

8. Pomegranate seeds: Both the seeds and the peel of pomegranates contain ellagitannins, which have anti-inflammatory effects on cells in the body.

9. Naturally occurring purple vegetables and fruit: Naturally purple-coloured foods, like red cabbage, aubergine (eggplant), beetroot, berries and plums, all contain compounds called anthocyanins. Studies are ongoing, so it's too early to say whether they are the daddies of the phytochemical world or not, but they have multiple benefits. Resveratrol, another antioxidant found in purple-coloured plant foods, is also thought to have potential anti-inflammatory activity.

10. Green leafy vegetables: Veggies like kale, Swiss chard (silverbeet), spinach and broccoli are packed with nutrients such as vitamins A, C, E and K, as well as plant-based omega-3s. All these nutrients have shown to be natural antioxidants and anti-inflammatory.

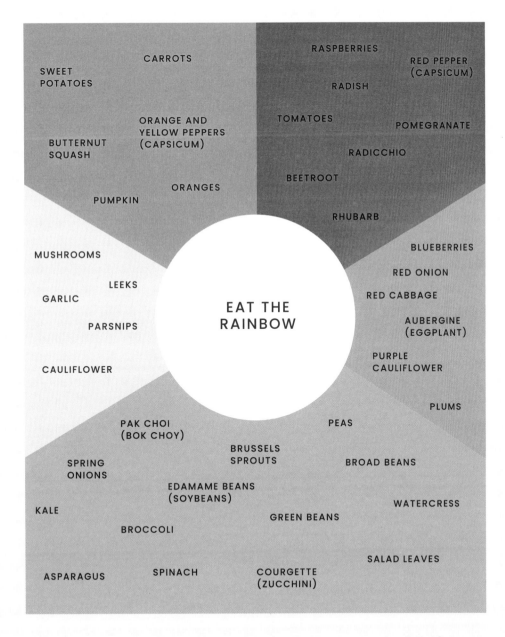

When Italians eat, they slow down and sit down. There is no multitasking, no mindless eating.

EAT LIKE YOU'RE ON THE MEDITERRANEAN

One diet that's considered anti-inflammatory is the Mediterranean diet. It's based on the traditional foods of the countries bordering the Mediterranean Sea, which include Italy, Spain, France and Greece. The principles of this diet are a good benchmark to guide you on your eating journey, and that's why a lot of my recipes have a Med-style influence. So, what does the Med diet look like?

1. Consistent balance. What's the real 'secret' to the Mediterranean diet? Consistently eating a balanced range of nutritious whole foods. Meals are built around seasonal vegetables and fruit, whole grains, beans and legumes, nuts and, of course, extra virgin olive oil. There are moderate amounts of dairy, poultry and eggs as well as seafood. Red meat is not excluded but it's eaten only occasionally. Sweet treats like gelato aren't eaten regularly, but they aren't forbidden. They are eaten as occasional treats (and usually with much pleasure). There are no 'good' or 'bad' foods. Rather, foods are seen on a spectrum of those to eat more and less of (see table opposite).

2. Home-cooked meals. Home-cooked meals are the norm in Mediterranean countries, and this has many health benefits. In the fast-paced world we live in, preparing meals at home has become less popular and takeaways and eating out has become the norm. You don't have to make everything from scratch; start where you are at. If you regularly buy ready meals, add some extra veggies or opt for those that are less ultra-processed. Next, if you buy ready-made pasta sauces, try making your own. Then build up to gradually making more home-cooked meals.

3. Eat in season. Buying local and eating in season is not only more economical, it's also better for your health. Seasonal produce is fresher, tastes better and usually has more nutrients. Frozen veggies and fruit are just as nutritious as their fresh counterparts, can be less expensive and are available all year around.

Eating seasonally also means you eat a wider variety of fresh produce, and by 'eating the rainbow', you maximise the variety of the phytonutrients you consume, which is important for maintaining a healthy microbiome (for more on this, see page 71).

4. Include herbs and spices. Mediterranean food is tasty, as it's flavoured with an abundance of herbs and spices, many of which contain active plant compounds that are thought to have strong anti-inflammatory properties. Herbs and spices are also excellent sources of antioxidants, so are a great way to boost overall health.

5. Eat mindfully. When I was doing my PhD in Milan, the whole research unit would stop for their lunch break and eat together. When I'm in London, there are hardly any days when I don't eat my lunch in a hurry at my computer. When Italians eat, they slow down and sit down. They look at their food, they smell their food, they talk about their food (there's lots of that!). There is no multitasking, no mindless eating. They just eat and enjoy! It's a lifestyle we should all adopt.

EAT MORE	EAT SOME	EAT LESS
Colourful vegetables (fresh and frozen)	White wheat products like white pasta (preferably al dente) and white rice (avoid sticky white rice)	Foods and drinks with added sugars
Whole fruit (fresh and frozen)		Fast food
Beans and lentils	Red meat	Ultra-processed foods
Whole grains	Saturated fat like butter or cheese	Processed meats
Plain yoghurts		Refined vegetable oils
Lean protein sources		
Unsalted nuts and seeds and nut butter		
Avocado		
Extra virgin olive oil		
Spices and herbs		

TAKEAWAYS

1. The relationship between the menopause and inflammation is not yet fully understood, however we know that women in the menopause are at increased risk of systemic inflammation.

2. Inflammation makes symptoms of the menopause worse and it further increases our risk of chronic diseases like type 2 diabetes, heart disease, arthritis and dementia.

3. Cooling inflammation is an essential part of a healthy menopause transition and following the Mediterranean diet is highly recommended.

4. Essentially, the Mediterranean way is a balanced diet that focuses on whole food. Meals are built around seasonal vegetables and fruit, whole grains, beans and legumes, nuts and, of course, extra virgin olive oil. There are moderate amounts of dairy, poultry and eggs as well as seafood. Red meat is not excluded but it is eaten occasionally. Fresh herbs and spices with strong anti-inflammatory properties are included in most meals.

5. The Mediterranean diet is more than a way of eating; it is a way of living. It's also important to remember that lifestyle habits (such as sleep, stress and activity levels) also play a role in inflammation.

Other nutrition areas to consider

Should you eat organic foods?

We still don't understand the impact of multiple exposure and bio-accumulation of pesticides and herbicides on health. We also don't know how different population groups are specifically affected, like menopausal women for example. However, some studies suggest the potential benefits of eating organic food are:

> **Lower pesticide and antibiotic residue.** Organically grown and reared produce will have less pesticides and antibiotics used on them than conventionally farmed products. Some pesticides and herbicides are known as endocrine disruptors. This means they may mess with your hormones.
> **More nutrients.** Organic products may have more antioxidants and flavonoids that offer the body protective benefits.
> **Higher omega-3 levels.** Higher amounts of omega-3s have been reported in organic meats, dairy and eggs as the food for organic livestock will have higher omega-3 levels.
> **Lower toxic metals.** Cadmium is a heavy metal that can be toxic. Studies show organic grains have lower cadmium levels than conventional grains, but this isn't the case for fruit and vegetables.

Points to consider include:

> The biggest barrier with going organic is cost. The first and most important point is that it is MUCH better to eat a variety of plant-based foods than to buy one organic packet of apples. The variety of foods will also lower your chances of exposure to a single pesticide. Buying in season and locally can also help lower your levels. Wash fresh fruit and vegetables well before eating them. My top foods to buy organic would be oats, berries, apples, spinach, lettuce, dairy products, poultry and meat.

Supplements

In an ideal world we would get all our vitamins and minerals from food. However, the reality is the 21st-century lifestyle poses challenges that increase the likelihood of us falling short of nutrients. In the menopause transition your body is more vulnerable. So, with that in mind, supplements have their place in helping to support your menopause journey. But they are not a substitute for good nutrition.

HOW TO USE SUPPLEMENTS

A big portion of my time with clients is spent discussing nutritional supplements: which ones they're taking, which ones actually work and which don't. Over the years, I have found some common themes.

Firstly, many women are taking a lot of supplements. I can see why. Many women are desperate for help and may have struggled to find the right support.

Secondly, some of the supplements women are taking are beneficial, but they are taking them in the wrong doses, at the wrong time or in the wrong cycles. They then get frustrated that the supplements don't work.

Thirdly, I see the placebo effect in action. There are some supplements that have very little scientific grounding, yet some women swear by them. The mind can be a powerful tool. If you expect something to work, it will most likely end up having a positive effect. If you want to consider using supplements, here are some tips:

1. Ensure you are using them safely. Check with your GP or doctor before taking any supplements if you have any medical conditions or are taking any medications as there may be contraindications or interactions.

2. Remember, more is not better. Just because something is good for you, doesn't mean you should take high doses of it, especially without checking with a health professional first.

3. If you think you would benefit from individual support, talk to a qualified registered health professional like a dietitian or registered nutritionist. They can help you decide which supplements may help and suggest appropriate dosages.

Here are some of the most common supplements, usually taken on their own or combined in a perimenopause/menopause supplement.

VITAMIN D

When you scan the body for vitamin D receptors you find them pretty much everywhere. This means it's a nutrient that not only supports our bones and immune system, it influences many other systems and may have multiple benefits for menopausal women. The UK government recommended adult vitamin D dosage is 400 IU (10mcg) per day when the sun is at its lowest (autumn and winter). Women with darker skin tones or gut issues such as inflammatory bowel disease may well need higher doses of up to 25mcg (1000 IU) or possibly more.

The science

As we go through menopause, we lose the protective effect of oestrogen on our bones, and vitamin D helps absorb calcium into our bones to keep them strong. Studies also show low levels of vitamin D affect mood, play a role in insulin resistance and lower sleep quality.

My verdict

I strongly suggest getting your vitamin D levels tested as it's an important one to get right; low levels can mimic early perimenopause. Optimal levels are 70-80nmol/L. Based on your bloods, you can get a supplement with the right dose.

OMEGA-3

Omega-3 fatty acids are essential fats that have anti-inflammatory properties. Recommendations vary from country to country, however most health organisations recommend an intake of at least 250–500 milligrams of combined EPA and DHA per day. The last dietary survey in the UK showed that, on average, we were getting around a third of that.

The science

The most positive research into omega-3s has been linked to their impact on mood and behaviour. Research into omega-3 and perimenopausal symptoms is limited but some studies suggest they may help reduce hot flushes and night sweats. Some studies link low levels of omega-3 to dry skin and hair.

My verdict

Eat some oily fish! If you're vegan, vegetarian or don't like fish, an omega-3 supplement can address a deficit and help to balance out high levels of omega-6 typically consumed in the Western diet (in ultra-processed food and refined oils). There isn't an agreed dosage for supplementation. In my practice, I recommend a 1-gram combined functional fatty acids (EPA and DHA) from fish oil. Vegans can opt for algae oil. According to the European Food Safety Authority, omega-3 fatty acid supplements can be safely consumed at doses of up to 5 grams per day. I recommend getting a blood test done to determine bespoke supplementation.

B VITAMINS

The eight B vitamins (B1, 2, 3, 5, 6, 7, 9 and 12) all have unique roles but work together to support and regulate energy, mood and cognitive function. Our B vitamin requirements increase with stress and alcohol consumption. Vitamin B12 is mainly found in animal products so it's recommended non-meat eaters take 10 micrograms of a B12 supplement per day.

The science

While there is limited research that looks specifically at B vitamins and menopause, there is some interesting research suggesting that B vitamins may help with hot flushes. More research is needed before we can draw firmer conclusions. Low levels of vitamin B6 have been found to impact progesterone production and have a negative impact on the immune and nervous systems.

My verdict

B vitamins are water soluble, which means they are not stored and should be consumed regularly. Some people find taking a B complex for a few weeks helps support their adrenal health when they are under pressure.

MAGNESIUM

Magnesium plays an important role in stress management and sleep as it works together with serotonin and melatonin, two neurotransmitters, to regulate mood and sleep. Both alcohol and stress use up your body's magnesium stores. Although it's widely available in food, according to the WHO, up to 95 per cent of the population is possibly deficient!

The science

There is limited research looking specifically at magnesium and menopause, however some studies suggest magnesium supplementation improves sleep duration and quality.

My verdict

For women in the menopause with anxiety, muscle aches, migraines, restless legs and sleep issues, magnesium supplements may help. The upper limit for magnesium supplements is 300–400 milligrams per day. There are different types of magnesium. If you want to try one, go for one that is a mixed formulation or magnesium glycinate as it's easily absorbed. I'm also a fan of Epsom salt in a warm bath.

PROBIOTICS

Probiotics are live microoganisms that, when consumed, help your body to maintain a healthy microbiome. You find them in fermented foods like bio-live yoghurt, kefir, kimchi, sauerkraut, miso and tempeh, or in nutritional supplements.

The science

If you eat fermented foods then, for most people, probiotic supplements are not necessary. The clinical data on supplementation with probiotics is mainly for use with a course of antibiotics, for irritable bowel syndrome (IBS) and traveller's diarrhoea. Research suggests that the bacterial composition of our mouths, vagina and gut can be altered by declining oestrogen levels. This may relate to perimenopausal symptoms including low mood, bloating and vaginal symptoms. There is some research suggesting that a lactobacillus-dominated vaginal microflora protects against changes in the vagina and a lactobacillus probiotic supplement may help to alleviate symptoms.

My verdict

Some women find a broad-spectrum probiotic (containing lactobacillus strains), aimed specifically at colonising the vaginal microbiome, helps prevent UTIs. If you want to try them, take them for eight to twelve weeks and keep a diary to see if your symptoms improve. They're safe for most people.

COLLAGEN

Collagen is the most abundant protein in the body. It's in bones, muscles, teeth, skin, tendons, cartilage, hair, nails, blood vessels and even the gut. As we age, our production slows and is lower quality. Most collagen powders are from animal sources.

The science

Hydrolysed collagen supplements are popular and the results look promising, particularly in relation to joint health and anti-aging, but the research is limited. They may help reduce joint pain from exercise or osteoarthritis. The research suggests you need to take them daily for at least eight to twelve weeks to see a result.

My verdict

If you can afford it, why not? There are currently no official guidelines on intake. Collagen is a safe supplement to take, with no recognised upper limit. If you take it, ensure it's good quality. If you're looking for long-lasting effects, you'll need to take it for a lifetime.

HERBAL SUPPLEMENTS AS ALTERNATIVES TO HRT

Women may consider taking herbal medicines alongside or instead of HRT. Many herbal supplements, such as black cohosh (*Cimicifuga racemosa*), red clover and maca (*Lepidium meyenii*), have been suggested for menopausal symptoms. However, the current scientific evidence for their effectiveness in relieving symptoms is either insufficient or generally weak.

If you want to try them, I recommend speaking to a registered herbalist (in the UK, this is through the National Institute of Medical Herbalists), who can guide you. If you're on prescription medications, always make sure you speak to your doctor.

When buying supplements, look out for a traditional herbal registration (THR) marking on the product packaging, which means it complies with quality standards relating to safety and manufacturing. Just because something is natural, doesn't mean it's safe.

PART 3

Living for success

For you to be the best version of yourself or to support your hormones, you need to think of your health in a holistic way.

My very first role, more than fifteen years ago, was working as a Sports Dietitian in a Human Performance Centre in the heart of London. I was part of a fantastic multidisciplinary team of medical doctors, exercise physiologists, biokineticists, psychologists, podiatrists, physiotherapists, osteopaths and strength and conditioning coaches. On top of that, we had specialist experts, like sleep and breathing experts, who popped in and out. The whole team worked together to optimise the performance potential of the client in front of us – whether they were a sporting athlete, a corporate leader or a stay-at-home mum. Having such a specialist team allowed us to look at an individual in a comprehensive way. Looking at a client through a holistic lens like this allowed each of us to identify areas that needed to be addressed and to implement targeted strategies that looked at the individual as a whole.

I very quickly learnt that no matter how good a performance nutritionist I was or how well my clients followed my recommendations, if they didn't spend enough time in bed, incorporate the correct movement mix, or work on their mindset, it would be a struggle for them to get the most out of their body.

For you to be your best version of yourself or to support your hormones, you need to think of your health in a holistic way. It's all connected.

Think about what you are likely to want to eat after you have only slept four hours. I know I would be feeling like ordering a nice pain au chocolat with a huge latte as my breakfast. And I'm not alone. For most of us, our sleep-deprived bodies would be craving fat, sugar and refined carbohydrates. Sleep affects your appetite and therefore your nutrition choices. Research shows that people who are sleep deprived eat an average of 300–400 more calories per day. And what you eat can influence how well you sleep. If you're struggling in one dimension of health, it usually means you'll be struggling in other areas too.

Now, here's the cool part. If the problems are connected, so are the solutions. Improving one dimension of your wellbeing can improve the others.

We have already acknowledged that the menopause transition can be tough and comes at a time when we are juggling other commitments, so we get sandwiched with pressure from above and below. Aging parents, teenagers, empty nesting, demanding career and so on. And we know it's a fact that your fluctuating hormones can make it harder to cope with everyday stress. If you don't take care, you become less resilient. Life can feel tougher.

In order to fully support you, we need to look at health through a holistic lens. We've covered nutrition in the previous section; now we're going to tackle the other three pillars of wellness:

> **sleep**
> **movement**
> **stress management.**

Sleep essentials

People will go to great lengths to ensure they have a nutrition plan, are taking their supplements and are following some sort of exercise program, yet they often forget about their sleep. But sleep is essential to health. I called it a pillar earlier; however it is actually the foundation of wellbeing. The other pillars all rest on sleep.

Chronic bad sleep does damage in the following ways.

> It makes it harder to lose weight and stay lean.
> Your skin suffers. 'Beauty sleep' is a real thing.
> It ages us faster. When we don't sleep, immune-regulating T-cells go down and inflammation goes up.
> It kills our mojo. While we sleep, we produce fresh neurotransmitters and regulate hormone production. Interference with this process affects emotional regulation, mood and stress management.
> It affects our rational decision-making. What we experience and learn gets cemented to memory while we sleep. Lack of sleep reduces alertness, impairs judgement and causes us to feel confused.
> It disrupts the balance in the gut microbiome for the worse.
> It increases our risk of chronic illnesses like type 2 diabetes and dementia.
> It disrupts our hormones, and is a big challenge for many women in the menopause transition.

There are many factors that affect our quality of sleep, some of which particularly affect women during the menopause.

- *Reduced progesterone levels. Progesterone plays a role in melatonin production, which helps you fall asleep.*
- *Low oestrogen levels can cause disruptive symptoms like night sweats and anxiety, which are further exacerbated by poor sleep. Oestrogen also helps you stay asleep, so low levels can mean disrupted sleep.*
- *Iron deficiency can lead to restless leg syndrome and insomnia.*
- *Joint pain.*
- *Bladder issues and getting up to use the loo.*
- *Sleep apnoea, which is a disorder that causes you to stop breathing at intervals while you sleep.*
- *Caffeine (a stimulant) still in circulation can impact your sleep.*
- *Alcohol can increase anxiety and night sweats and directly impacts the quality of your sleep (more on that later).*
- *A snoring partner (a big cause for divorce!).*
- *Children who wake you up.*
- *Prescription medications or over-the-counter drugs.*

This may feel like an overwhelming list, but rest assured there are strategies you can put in place to fix things. This is super important as a healthy menopause starts by getting really good in bed!

Know how much sleep you need

All adults should be aiming to get at least seven hours of sleep a night.

Entire books have been written on sleep, so I will keep it simple and succinct. Knowing how much sleep you need every night is a good place to start. Most people need seven to nine hours of sleep per night. Seven should be your baseline. Ideally, that's seven hours when you are actually asleep. You therefore need to factor in transition sleep when you're thinking about going to bed. Stopping what you are doing at 10.29pm and expecting to be out cold by 10.30pm is very unlikely. You need to start heading in the direction of bed by 10pm.

There is a common myth that people over 60 need less sleep. Many older adults do have a hard time getting the sleep they need, however this doesn't mean they need less sleep. All adults should be aiming to get at least seven hours of sleep a night.

The best way to gauge where in the seven-to-nine-hours spectrum you function best is to spend a week or so noting down how much sleep you think you are getting and then reflecting on how you feel. Do you feel better after 7.5 hours than at seven? Do you wake up naturally before nine hours?

Every credible piece of research demonstrates that you pay a big price in terms of short-term performance and productivity and your risk of diseases if you consistently get less than seven hours a night. In fact, studies show that after two nights of not sleeping more than seven hours, your body goes into high-alert mode. An abundance of cortisol, the stress hormone, is released. A practical and perhaps realistic tip is if it's a real struggle to get your seven to nine hours of sleep every night, try to at least prioritise getting seven to nine hours every third night as damage control.

Sleep debt results from getting less than seven hours of sleep each night. Sleep debt is cumulative, meaning the more nights with less sleep you get, the more you feel the negative effects. If we don't address the sleep debt, we break. Professor Matthew Walker, the sleep guru, says it as bluntly as 'the shorter your sleep, the shorter your life'. The good news is you can catch up on sleep. Napping or sleeping in on the weekends can help you catch up on sleep, but it can take several days to recover from the negative effects of sleep loss. The best strategy is to minimise your risk of getting into sleep debt by prioritising sleep.

DIFFERENT TYPES OF SLEEP

There are two essential types of sleep: non-rapid eye movement (NREM) and rapid eye movement (REM) sleep or light sleep. NREM sleep is deep and restorative, allowing you to feel more rested in the morning. REM is lighter sleep that allows your body to do the emotional processing it needs. When you are asleep, you cycle from NREM to REM approximately every 90 minutes. Ensuring you get enough of the different stages of sleep (sleep quality) is important, however the first step is to ensure you are getting enough sleep (sleep duration).

How to sleep soundly

Solution time. Here are some tools that form part of your menopause toolkit.

GOOD SLEEP HYGIENE

If you've ever had kids, you'll know all too well the importance of creating a bedtime routine. Your body needs transition time and environmental cues to wind down. This is referred to as sleep hygiene. Try this:

1. Dim the lights in the evenings, particularly the hour before bed.

2. Turn off electrical devices at least 60 minutes before bed. Devices stimulate our brain, blocking the release of your sleep hormone. If you really must look at dog videos or the headlines on the internet (I am guilty of this too!), consider getting blue-light-blocking glasses. But better still, get yourself a paper book.

3. Keep your bedroom cool. Your body needs to drop its core temperature by about one degree to initiate sleep and stay asleep during the night. The optimal temperature for a bedroom is 18–22 degrees Celsius (about 68 degrees Fahrenheit). So, turn off the radiator, open the window or get yourself a fan. Having a warm bath or shower before bed can also help as your body temperature will drop after this.

4. Keep your bedroom dark and quiet. Investing in shutters or blackout blinds is a good idea. An eye mask does the job too. If noise is an issue or you are a light sleeper, ear plugs can help. Some people find a white noise machine can help too.

DESIGN BETTER DAYS FOR BETTER NIGHTS

Restful sleep has as much to do with what you do in your day as it does with what you do at night. Eat to optimise your blood glucose. Just as not getting enough sleep affects blood-sugar levels, fluctuating blood-sugar levels also affect sleep quality. Hydrating well throughout your day means that you don't need to drink gallons of water before you go to bed. Minimising stimulants like nicotine and caffeine, especially later in the day, is key. Even though alcohol feels as though it's relaxing, it isn't; it massacres deep sleep. Try this:

1. When you wake up, get some natural daylight as soon as possible. A 20-minute walk outside is ideal.

2. Do you wake to pee? Limit fluids to two hours before bedtime. Drinking too much liquid before bed can cause you to wake in the night to go to the loo. You don't want interrupted sleep.

3. Experiment to see how much caffeine is too much and what your cut-off time is. Caffeine stays in the body for at least six hours. If you are struggling with your sleep and still want to have a hot drink at 4pm, opt for a decaffeinated choice. If you're feeling anxious, you may want to ease up on the caffeine.

4. Be mindful of how much and how often you drink alcohol, particularly if you sleep badly or are anxious. While it may help you to fall asleep, alcohol can disrupt the sleep cycle and decrease sleep quality.

Your body clock does best with a relatively consistent bedtime and wake-up time.

BE CONSISTENT

Your body clock loves a routine and does best with a relatively consistent bedtime and wake-up time, even on the weekend. While it may take time to establish this sort of routine, it's what you need to aim for. Based on our circadian rhythms, some sleep experts also say that in restorative terms, every hour of sleep before midnight is worth two hours after. Try this:

1. Head in the direction of bed at least 30 minutes before you want to be asleep.

2. Try to go to bed and wake up at the same time every day. While this may be unrealistic seven days a week, try to be as consistent as possible.

3. If bedtime slips, try to anchor the waking time as it helps regulate when you go to bed the following day.

4. Develop a bedtime routine that is relaxing and becomes familiar. Watching Netflix in bed is not sleep friendly. Some stretching, breathing, meditation or just reading a trashy magazine is.

5. Try to get into bed at least an hour before midnight or sooner if you can.

DO A BRAIN DUMP

We have all been there. You're in bed, the lights are out, you should be asleep, yet you are staring at the ceiling with your mind looping, thinking about all the things on your to-do list for tomorrow, tossing and turning and getting more and more stressed as you know you should be asleep. Research shows that if you write out a list of whatever is on your mind before going to bed, you're less likely to stay up thinking about it. Try this:

1. Keep a notepad and pen by your bed and write down the things on your mind: emails you need to reply to, calls you need to make, which child needs a PE outfit, creative ideas, the things you should have said and so on. It's a brain dump, which science shows clears your mind.

2. In the morning, review the list, as that way your brain knows you are looking at it and will soon get out of the routine of trying to remember it overnight.

PREPARE FOR THOSE NIGHT SWEATS

About 75 per cent of women in the Western world experience night sweats. If you fall into that group, be proactive and try to minimise the negative impact of the sweats on your sleep. Try this:

1. Keep a spare set of pyjamas or a little towel beside your bed. This way, when you get woken up soaked you are prepared for a quick change into something dry and can then get back into bed.

2. Consider trying cooling sheets and pillows. There are all sorts of products to try that are cooling, lightweight and breathable. They could be made out of linen, bamboo fibres or microfibres. While they may not completely cure your sleep problems, they may solve part of the puzzle.

3. Sleep with a fan. It keeps the room cool and doubles as a white noise machine. Perfect if your partner's (or the dog's) snoring also keeps you up.

The role of alcohol in poor sleep

While you can drink during the menopause, there are many reasons why it might be worth keeping an eye on how much and how often you are drinking. Menopause and alcohol are not the best combination.

While you may think a glass of wine makes you feel drowsy initially, you will pay for it in the second half of the night. Alcohol affects your REM sleep, which is when most of the emotional processing occurs. As alcohol levels drop during the night, your brain goes into rebound arousal, where you may toss and turn and experience more vivid and stressful dreams. This means you are likely to wake up more regularly. Alcohol is also a diuretic, which means you will be doing more bathroom runs than normal.

Alcohol not only affects the quality of your sleep, it also negatively impacts weight, digestive issues, mood, brain fog and hot flushes. Current recommendations are to drink no more than fourteen units per week. According to many experts, this is the lower limit rather than the upper limit. The less you drink, the better. Higher levels of alcohol are linked to cancers like breast cancer as well as fatty liver and cardiovascular disease.

It's easy to lose track of how much you are drinking, so keep in mind the following:

> A unit of alcohol is 10ml of pure alcohol but this depends on the strength and size of your drink
> One shot (25ml) of spirits at 40 per cent = 1 unit
> A medium (175ml) glass of 12 per cent wine = about 2 units
> A pint (568ml) of standard beer at 5.2 per cent = 3 units
> Cocktails = generally around 2.5 units
> A bottle of wine (at 13.5 per cent) = 10 units.

Movement

Did you know that after smoking, not moving enough (i.e. being sedentary) is rated as one of the major contributors to poor health? And movement matters even more during the menopause transition.

But what I see from many of my clients is that movement can be tricky. Even if they know it's good for them, it's often one of the first things that goes when they are time poor. Add to it the fact that their fluctuating hormones may affect their energy levels and mood, and their aching joints and muscles also make them feel like exercise is the last thing they want to do.

Let's start by understanding exactly why you need to make movement part of your lifestyle. No matter what your current relationship with exercise is like, it's never too late to start.

Why movement matters

Apart from keeping in shape, movement offers many other benefits, especially in the menopause years.

> **Improves quality of life.** Movement boosts your mood. When you exercise, it increases endorphins, which are brain chemicals associated with feeling happy, less anxious and more confident.
> **Supports good sleep.** Specifically, moderate to vigorous exercise can help reduce the time it takes to fall asleep, improve how well you sleep and decrease the amount of time you lie awake in bed during the night.

> **Prevents weight gain.** Women tend to lose muscle mass and gain fat around their middle in the perimenopause. Regular physical activity helps prevent weight gain and supports a healthier body shape.
> **Helps manage hot flushes** by improving the control and stability of the systems in your body involved in temperature and heat dissipation.
> **Strengthens your bones.** The menopause increases your risk of developing osteoporosis. Exercise, particularly resistance exercise, helps to strengthen the bones, slows down bone loss and therefore reduces your risk of fractures and osteoporosis.
> **Supports a healthy microbiome.** The more you move, the happier your gut bacteria are. And it appears that the positive changes from movement are different to the effects induced by diet. Researchers have found that if you are sedentary, then you exercise for six weeks, you get a significant increase in gut bacteria, which assists in the production of short-chain fatty acids that prevent metabolic diseases such as diabetes. But when you stop exercising, your gut health returns to its sluggish self and you are no longer protected. Don't over exercise, as too much can be detrimental to your gut, causing it to become 'leakier'.
> **Reduces risk of heart disease and type 2 diabetes.** Exercise helps your whole body to become and remain healthier, which helps counter the increased risk of diseases like heart disease, diabetes and certain types of cancer that come with the menopause.

How much should I be moving?

When it comes to exercise, the first and most important place to start is with a concept known as non-exercise activity thermogenesis (NEAT). This is a fancy way of describing movement that is part of your day-to-day life. Essentially, it's how much you walk. Walking is a very underrated form of exercise. The more steps you take, the better, as this helps keep your metabolism activated and your muscles awake. You can use your phone or any device to track your steps. There is debate around exactly how many steps you need to do, but a good ballpark to aim for is 10,000.

STAND MORE, SIT LESS

I often work from home, and on those days I have found that if I'm not proactive, I only do about 500 steps a day tops. So, last year I decided to invest in a standing desk. It was a game changer for my body and my mood. Sitting down for long periods can tighten your muscles and cause tightness in your hips and back. Standing also burns more calories than sitting, even if you are standing still. The difference is not massive but over time it could add up.

PLAN TO MOVE

The other thing we need to incorporate into our days is structured or planned movement. It's recommended that we do at least 150 minutes of moderate activity a week or 75 minutes of vigorous-intensity activity a week. Let's break this down for you to make it practical.

1. A mix of different types of activity is important. So, get some cardio in, but also some flexibility and strength work (or what we call functional strength – super-important for perimenopausal women). This doesn't mean you have to lift heavy weights; it just means you need to exert yourself. And it's good to do this in ways that are functional. So, rather than just doing a static lunge, do walking lunges. Rather than doing a bicep curl, do a movement that is more like picking something up from the floor and placing it on a top shelf. The important thing is to start from where you are.

2. Spread your activity evenly over four to five days a week or every day. Don't just go for it on the weekend. Some women might find they need more rest days; if this is you, you can intersperse them throughout the week.

3. You can achieve your weekly target with several short sessions of very vigorous-intensity activity or a mix of moderately vigorous and very vigorous-intensity activity.

4. Incorporate some high-intensity interval training (HIIT). Research shows that perimenopausal women don't benefit from long hours of steady-state cardio but get more benefit from a high-intensity interval style of training. But start small and build up slowly. You can join a fitness class, find a trainer or training buddy. YouTube is a fantastic resource to tap into for inspiration.

5. Make movement enjoyable as you are more likely to stick to it in the long term. So, find your thing and build it into your life.

What type of movement should I be doing?

To keep your bones strong, you need to do both muscle-strengthening and weight-bearing exercise.

There is a common perception among women that we need to be doing loads of cardio to 'burn' fat. This is wrong. Actually, we need to do strength training to maximise muscle mass. Our declining hormones mean we are more at risk of losing muscle mass. However, another important reason to do strength training is for our bones. Muscles and bones are intricately linked, so you need to strengthen your muscles too as this supports your bones.

We want strong bones to minimise our long-term risk of osteoporosis. Around 10 per cent of a woman's bone mass is lost in the first five years of the menopause and this increases your risk of osteoporosis, a condition where your bones are more likely to break. To keep your bones strong, you need to do both muscle-strengthening and weight-bearing exercise.

WEIGHT-BEARING EXERCISE

Weight-bearing exercise is any activity where you support your body weight through your feet and legs (or arms and hands). So, with one or two feet on the ground, your bones and muscles are working against gravity. Swimming, for example, is not weight bearing. Walking, climbing stairs, jogging, hiking, gardening, playing tennis, dancing and exercise classes are all weight-bearing activities. For exercise to benefit our bones, it needs to be weight-bearing exercise as this stimulates the process of reinforcing the protein mesh and its mineralisation.

RESISTANCE EXERCISE

Resistance or muscle-strengthening exercise is where you move your muscles against some resistance, like lifting weights, using rubber bands or doing body-weight exercises like push-ups. To get health benefits from strength work, you should do it to the point where you need a short rest before repeating the activity. There are many ways you can strengthen your muscles, whether you are at home or in a gym.

Examples of muscle-strengthening activities include:

> carrying heavy shopping bags
> yoga
> Pilates
> tai chi
> lifting weights
> working with resistance bands
> doing exercises that use your own body weight such as push-ups and the plank
> heavy gardening such as digging and shovelling.

Managing stress

We have seen the effects that hormonal decline during perimenopause can have on our physical health, but it can have a profound impact on our mental health too. The impact is often underestimated. Because menopause itself is stressful for our body, the link between stress and menopause can sometimes feel like a negative feedback loop. Feeling low, depressed, invisible, unheard, empty, flat and not recognising the reflection in the mirror will have a knock-on effect on every sphere of life – relationships, family life, work, you name it.

Managing stress is a critical part of your menopause toolkit as there is not a single symptom that isn't improved by calming your nervous system. Weight gain, brain fog, hot flushes, mood, food sensitivities, sleep issues, low libido, headaches and so on – all of them can be improved by calming your nervous system.

Let's understand stress

There is good and bad stress. When stress is good, you feel alive and you thrive. You learn new things. Take the example of me writing this book. I had a deadline to meet. This motivated me to hit the laptop and boosted my brain to focus. A work deadline or presentation are examples of good stress. They drive you to up your performance. An important part of remaining in this zone is ensuring you build in daily rest and recovery time.

So, when does stress become a problem? The Yerkes-Dodson stress curve below illustrates this nicely.

It shows there is an optimal amount of pressure where you thrive. When the level of stress becomes too high, not only do you start to freak out, it begins to take a toll on your body. In nervous system terms, you have an overactive sympathetic nervous system. If you are in this mode for a sustained period of time, your body suffers.

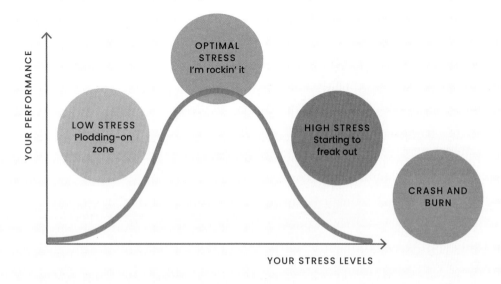

Stress that lasts for days, weeks or months without any recovery time is chronic stress and really takes a toll.

Physically, you start to crave unhealthy food. Your nights are full of interrupted sleep, especially early-morning waking. You feel more bloated. You may suffer from heartburn or heart palpitations. You catch every cold or bug that's going around. Your libido tanks. You are excessively anxious. You feel low. It's hard to focus or you experience brain fog more. No matter what you do, you seem to be gaining weight around the middle. Ironically, a lot of these symptoms mirror general symptoms of the perimenopause.

CHRONIC STRESS

Stress that lasts for days, weeks or months without any recovery time is chronic stress and really takes a toll. Think of yourself as a bucket with two taps. One tap fills the bucket up with water, and one lets water drain out. Chronic stress can drain our bucket. Recovery fills the bucket back up.

The aim of the game is to always have something in the bucket. To do this, you need to try to fill it as much as you drain it. The stress-bucket analogy was developed in 2002 by Professor Alison Brabban and Dr Douglas Turkington to help people think about their tolerance to life stresses. The size of your bucket is a product of your genes, your personality and life experiences. We are all different. While we may not be able to change the size of the bucket, we can develop coping strategies to fill our bucket more than we drain it.

Things that can drain your bucket can generally be grouped into four main areas:

> **Emotional stress:** Strained relationships, financial burdens, work stress, being a carer, bereavements, phobias.

> **Food stress:** Not eating enough (i.e. fad diets) or poor nutrition (particularly unbalanced blood-sugar levels).
> **Environmental and lifestyle stress:** Smoking, poor sleep, sedentary lifestyle, alcohol or drug use, environmental toxins in household products and toiletries.
> **Physical stress:** Overexertion, injury or illness.

If we go back to thinking about your nervous system for a moment, when you are stressed, your fight-or-flight sympathetic nervous system is activated. There is another part of your nervous system called the parasympathetic nervous system. Its main role is to control automatic functions in your body, like breathing, your heartbeat and digestion. However, it also has an important connection between your mind and your body through a nerve called the vagus nerve. The role of the vagus nerve is to help tone down your sympathetic nervous system, giving the body a sense of balance and calm.

If you use any wearable devices, like the Whoop fitness tracker, Oura ring or Garmin watch, they measure your heart rate variability (HRV), which is a measure of how well your vagus nerve is working. These measurements are not entirely accurate but they do give you a good indication. A higher HRV is generally considered an indicator of a healthy heart, improved psychological wellbeing and quality of life. HRV levels change naturally from day to day based on the level of activity, work-related stress and amount of rest you get. Genetic factors play a big role in HRV, so comparison to others' HRV numbers is meaningless.

The amazing thing is that there are basic healthy living strategies that can help activate your vagus nerve, allowing your body to keep calm. And these vagus-stimulating strategies are a way of ensuring your bucket is being filled up, that you recover, build resilience and are looking after yourself.

How to fill up your bucket and manage your stress

While I will be sharing some self-care strategies, please don't take these as a prescription, but more as ideas and inspiration to dabble with. You need to figure out what fits your needs and goals. The menopause is absolutely the time to be looking after you – find YOUR way of doing just that.

Once you find your way, develop rituals. Build them into your daily plan. There are places in the world called blue zones where people live the longest, happy and healthy lives. Many people in these zones arrive at 100 years old active, healthy and with a sense of purpose.

A key aspect of blue-zone living is that residents build good habits into their lifestyles, so it becomes a way of living. They follow generally healthy, balanced diets and move regularly but don't over-exercise. Dancing is a common theme. It brings together movement and connection and it's fun! They also prioritise sleep.

For more ideas, try the following:

BUILD A SWITCHING-OFF ROUTINE INTO YOUR DAILY SCHEDULE

How do you unwind and disconnect? Leisure activities like listening to music, cooking, playing board games, watching movies or TV shows, or reading books give us something enjoyable to do while helping take our minds off stressful situations. Find your thing.

TALK IT OUT

Research shows that offloading what is on your mind, whether with your partner, a trusted friend or a family member, can really help you manage stress. Working with a therapist or a coach also helps provide perspective on difficult situations and allows you to develop coping strategies in a safe environment. Cognitive behavioural therapy (CBT) is a particularly effective intervention for challenging unhelpful thoughts and feelings.

WRITE IT OUT

Personally, I find journalling a good starting-off point in trying to help unravel the big ball of interwoven thoughts and feelings. Research shows it is linked to decreased mental distress and improved mood.

GET CREATIVE!

Expressing yourself through activities like drawing, painting, playing music and crafting can effectively reduce stress.

CONNECT

We are human beings. This means that we thrive on connection. Studies show that people who feel more connected to others have lower levels of anxiety and depression and higher levels of self-esteem and empathy. Connection

Make room for connections. Let go of relationships that are not serving you.

could be speaking with a stranger, doing something nice for your neighbours, joining a group of like-minded people linked with your hobby or faith, finding and working with a mentor you look up to, catching up with an old friend or asking a loved one for a hug. Make room for connections. Let go of relationships that are not serving you. Invest in those that do. Find your tribe. Build a support network.

SPEAK KINDLY TO YOURSELF

The way you speak to yourself matters. When our inner dialogue sounds more like a bully than a best friend, the impact is the same. We live with that voice 24 hours a day, seven days a week. Notice your inner voice. How do you speak to yourself? Speak kindly to yourself. Become your best cheerleader.

BREATHE

Breathing helps to bring you to the present. In general, for vagus nerve activation, breathing is a good place to start as many of us don't breathe properly. Insane, right? There are breath specialists who run breathwork courses and many apps like Just Breathe or Calm include breathing. However, why not just pause? Stop and take a deep breath in. And out. Do this more throughout your day.

MEDITATE

Mindfulness and meditation are practices that bring your awareness to your thoughts and feelings without attachment or judgement. Find a class. Immerse yourself in it by booking a holiday that focuses on this. Or start slowly with the support of apps like Headspace, Insight Timer, Calm or Buddhify. Activities like yoga and tai chi include meditation.

PRACTISE MINDFULNESS

Being fully present. For some, this may be meditation, but it could be any activity that gets you to tap into all your senses to bring you into the present. It could also be mindfully making a cup of tea, dancing to a song and getting 100 per cent absorbed in the beat of the music, going for a walk and noticing the leaves, sounds and colours and the world around you. Or you could sign up for a mindfulness-based stress-reduction program with a professional to guide you.

GET OUTSIDE

Mother nature is healing. It has many calming effects that help us feel more relaxed. If you can't get to a forest or a park, go outside in your garden or yard if you have one.

BE SPONTANEOUS

Be open to sometimes doing things off schedule, off the cuff and going with the flow. Studies suggest it can be beneficial to our emotional health. It could help you to connect to your playful inner child, be more creative and build up your resilience.

TRY COLD THERAPIES

Research is increasingly showing that cold therapy (sea swimming, ice baths, plunge pools, cryotherapy or even cold showers) improves our response to stress and enables the body to become more resistant to stress.

FIND PURPOSEFUL ACTIVITIES

Having a sense of purpose is important as it's linked with a sense of identity and improved overall mental health. It will help motivate you and make you feel fulfilled.

Your menopause lifestyle toolkit

I want this book to serve as a valuable guide that you can go back to as your menopause journey ebbs and flows. I also want to arm you with practical tools to empower you. With that in mind, I want to give you a toolbox of practical ideas that you can use to help you deal with your symptoms and support your menopause journey. Remember, you are an active participant in your health, so now is the time to take hold of the reins. Invest in the time to put your toolkit together before the symptoms hit. If they have already hit, use the tips to do some damage control. It's never too late!

I have focused on the main pain points I hear from the women I support. Go through the list and highlight the ones that resonate with you. See how the suggested tips can fit into your world. With all of these tips, remember you are aiming for progress, not perfection. Perfection doesn't exist. None of the tips will make you feel like a superwoman in an instant, either. Think about what a 'little better' might look like, even if it's by one or two notches. It will be a little trial and error. It's about building small steps and changes in your life that nudge you in the direction you want to go and that will stick, not just for five days, but for months and years to come.

If any of these areas don't resonate or appeal, or you find them triggering, that's okay. Skip the section and come back to it when you're ready. If you need some more support as you work things out, then check out the information on page 255.

Managing your weight

Menopause weight gain is a struggle for many women. It isn't all about aesthetics; being overweight increases your risk of chronic diseases like type 2 diabetes and high blood pressure.

THINK SLOW AND STEADY

Rapid weight loss is not sustainable. Healthy weight loss, where you protect your muscle and lose predominantly fat mass, is when you lose 0.5–1 kilogram or 1–2 pounds a week. I recommend finding an objective way to monitor your progress. This doesn't mean becoming obsessed with numbers. Numbers don't define you. However, it's useful to know where you're starting from and it's a way to track your progress. Know the number on the scale but know other numbers too. What is your waist circumference? How many vegetables did you eat yesterday? How many plant points (see page 67) have you had this week?

There are so many ways to lose weight. It's about finding a way that works and feels good for you. I recommend maintaining a balanced diet overall, upping your veggies, prioritising protein and including some of the healthier carbs and some fat (for more, see page 56). The key is to keep an eye on your portions (see page 60). Putting down your fork between bites, chewing your food properly and savouring your meals helps you connect with feelings of fullness, which can help to manage overeating. Practise what the Japanese call *hara hachi bu*, or eating until you are

You are an active participant in your health, so now is the time to take hold of the reins.

80 per cent full. Keep at least ten to twelve hours between dinner and breakfast.

FLUIDS BEFORE MEALS

It's easy to mistake dehydration for hunger. Ghrelin, the hunger hormone, is released when your stomach is empty. Having a glass of water before a meal or a soup to start is a great way to manage your appetite as it can temporarily turn off ghrelin.

UNDERSTAND THE TYPES OF HUNGER

Hunger is your physiological need for food, whereas appetite is your desire for food. Before you begin eating, try to check in with how your body is feeling. How hungry are you? Are you eating because you are physically hungry or is it out of boredom or anxiety?

Being severely hungry before a meal can make it difficult to slow down and eat mindfully. Commit to incorporating balanced meals throughout the day so you aren't ravenous at mealtimes.

Recognise when you are eating for reasons other than physical hunger. If you have emotional hunger, try non-food solutions like journalling, changing your environment, taking a short walk, practising deep breathing or calling a loved one or a professional.

SNACK SMART

For the majority of people in the Western world, snacks contribute to 20 per cent of our daily calorie intake, so it's important we plan for them. A healthy snack contains some fibre, as well as some protein or healthy fats. For snack inspiration, go to page 152.

EAT STARCHY CARBS AT THE RIGHT TIME

Opt for low-glycaemic index (slow release) carbs that are whole foods or whole grains, as well as vegetables and fruit. Eat your starchy carbohydrates earlier in the day, at breakfast and lunch. Serve up the right carb portion sizes (see page 51).

CONSIDER A BOOZE BREAK

The 'beer belly' isn't a myth! Drinking too much alcohol encourages fat to be stored as visceral fat around the abdomen. The calories in alcohol are plentiful and 'empty'. A bottle of wine contains 750 calories but offers the body nothing else. Alcohol can also change the way your body burns fat as it's more focused on breaking down the alcohol than metabolising any of the other calories you consume. This encourages those excess calories to be stored as visceral fat. Alcohol also lowers willpower, making in-the-moment decisions like 'chicken salad or burger and fries' much harder. Reduce your alcohol intake or consider a booze break. See the drinks section (page 240) for alcohol alternatives.

WALK MORE

Movement in your day (non-exercise activity thermogenesis or NEAT) keeps your metabolism boosted. Park further from the office or get off a bus stop earlier. Take the stairs instead of the lift. Monitor your steps. Aim for an average of ten thousand steps a day. Two thousand extra steps a week is a good incremental increase.

ADDRESS YOUR STRESS

Stress puts your body into survival mode, which means fat loss is not a priority. Find ways to stimulate your vagus nerve as this allows your body to calm down. Some breathing exercises are a great place to start.

KEEP A FOOD DIARY

Keep a daily log of what you eat and drink and how it makes you feel to give insight into your eating habits and potential food sensitivities. You can also take it to a dietitian or registered nutritionist for their input.

Coping with hot flushes

Approximately 75 per cent of women in the Western world experience hot flushes. Typically, they begin in the late perimenopause phase, however for some women, they do not begin until after menopause. Hot flushes are almost always due to menopause. They can be stressful and can negatively impact work and sleep.

STAY HYDRATED

Not drinking enough water can put your body thermostat further out of whack, which can make hot flushes worse. Carry a water bottle with you at all times.

EAT TO BALANCE YOUR BLOOD SUGAR

Hot flushes and night sweats are influenced by your blood-sugar levels. Low blood sugars are thought to trigger hot flushes. Constantly high blood-sugar levels increase your risk of weight gain. Extra weight is linked with higher frequency and severity of hot flushes. Have balanced, regular meals. For more information about how to balance your plate, see page 60.

EAT MORE PLANT OESTROGENS

Phytoestrogens are plant-based compounds that have weak oestrogen-like effects on the body that can reduce hot flushes. Although the research into their effectiveness is mixed and appears to vary between individuals, it's worth a try. Minimally processed soy-based foods like tofu, soy milk, edamame beans or soy yoghurt are the highest in phytoestrogens. However, lignans, found in flaxseeds, are also a brilliant daily addition. It's better to get phytoestrogens from food than a supplement. It can take two or three months to see the benefits.

GO EASY ON THE CAFFEINE

Caffeine intake and hot flushes is not a well-researched area, however some studies have linked caffeine with an increased severity of hot flushes. Caffeine sensitivity varies between individuals. Try a decaffeinated drink and see if you notice a difference after a week or so. If cutting out caffeine is unrealistic, be mindful of when and how much you have (see page 42).

BE PREPARED

The many triggers for hot flushes range from spicy foods, hot drinks, alcohol, changes in temperature, heavy clothing and stress, to use of appliances like hairdryers. Know your triggers so you can put strategies in place. If exercise sets off a hot flush, dress in light, breathable clothing, position yourself in front of a fan when you work out or buy a mini portable fan to take to classes. Cooling facial sprays are also fantastic.

MANAGE STRESS

It's common for a hot flush to come on when you're nervous or anxious. Nurture your ability to stay grounded. Learn deep breathing techniques or start regular meditation or mindfulness practice. Some early research points to

Approximately 75 per cent of women in the Western world experience hot flushes.

mindfulness meditation and hypnotherapy being helpful in managing hot flushes.

CUT BACK ON ALCOHOL

Alcohol causes your blood vessels to dilate, which can trigger a hot flush. Although all alcohol will do this, many women find that red wine is the biggest culprit. Ideally, you should try to switch to non-alcohol alternatives (see page 240), particularly if you're going through a stressful period. If you really want your glass of wine, water it down with lots of ice or sparkling water. Try white wine instead of red.

HAVE A COLD SHOWER

This is an instant relief to calm a hot flush. Dabbling with cold-water immersion (cold-water swimming or ice baths), cryotherapy or simply having cold showers daily will also help stimulate your 'feel-good' dopamine hormone. Mix things up. New experiences and unexpected surprises release more dopamine.

Increase your energy

It's normal to feel tired from time to time, but if you're tired of being tired (i.e. the menopause fatigue), you need to work on boosting your energy levels.

KEEP YOUR WATER BOTTLE NEARBY

Dehydration slows circulation and affects the flow of oxygen throughout the body and brain, making you feel tired, sluggish and less focused. Drink a glass of water first thing in the morning. Sip from your water bottle regularly throughout the day. Use alarms or notifications to keep you accountable.

Swap sugary drinks for sparkling water with slices of orange or cucumber or try my switches from page 240.

SUGAR CRAVINGS?

These are caused by many factors. It could be not enough sleep, stress or mild dehydration. You could be low on protein or you may need to unshackle yourself from refined carbohydrates. Keep a food diary to give you more insight into your habits.

When we have low energy, it's tempting to reach for that sugary boost. However, this will only fuel the blood-sugar roller-coaster ride. You may want to go cold turkey and cut out all added sugar for a period before you reintroduce small amounts. Or you may just want to make small changes to help you cut down on your intake without you noticing it too much. Stop adding sugar to tea, coffee and hot drinks. Remember, honey and maple syrup are sugar too. Sweeten porridge and cereal with fresh fruit or dried figs. Swap fruit-flavoured yoghurts for natural yoghurt and add your own fruit. Be wary of 'sugar-free' foods. They contain artificial sweeteners which still taste sweet and continue to feed your sweet tooth. Switch refined options like white rice or bread to wholegrain. Swap milk chocolate for dark (more than 70 per cent cocoa).

BE SMART WITH PORTIONS

As a rough guide, you should have half a plate of vegetables, a fistful of protein, wholegrain carbs and a portion of healthy fat at breakfast and lunch. At dinner, if you are in weight-loss mode, load up with veggies.

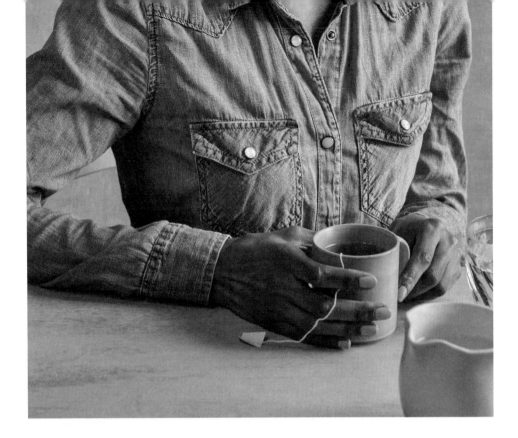

DO SOME MEAL PREP

Healthy eating is more likely to happen if you're prepared. Find a routine that works and stick to it. Knowing exactly when you'll shop for groceries and prepare your meals will help you form a good routine. Come up with a menu. Build a shopping list from that. This will help you to be as efficient as possible when you hit the supermarket and you will be less tempted to buy random items (your wallet will thank you, too).

GET MOVING

Although it's probably the last thing you feel like doing, movement is exactly what you need to increase your energy levels. Go for a walk. Do a two-minute plank when you watch the news and ten star jumps as the kettle boils. Find ways to move more.

HONOUR REST

Prioritise your sleep. If you don't sleep enough, you will have low energy and a reduced desire to exercise. Even an extra 30 minutes a night can make a difference. Make sure you head in the direction of bed well before you want to be asleep.

CONSIDER A B VITAMIN SUPPLEMENT

B vitamins support the body to produce chemicals that affect mood and other brain functions. You may want to consider supplementing with a B-complex daily for a couple of weeks to help support your adrenals and boost your energy levels.

Boost brain function

Your brain is kind of a big deal. It's in charge of keeping your heart beating and your lungs breathing, and allows you to move, think and feel. Seventy per cent of women report mood changes in the menopause transition.

PRIORITISE HYDRATION
Water helps carry nutrients to your brain, helps your brain cells communicate with each other and clears out toxins and waste that impair brain function. If you're dehydrated, your brain doesn't work as well. Don't wait until you're thirsty; sip water steadily throughout the day. Eat plenty of water-rich fruit and vegetables like courgette (zucchini), cucumbers, leafy greens, tomatoes, radishes and berries.

CONTROL BLOOD SUGAR
The brain is the most energy-demanding organ, using up 20 per cent of your body's energy. If your blood-sugar levels fluctuate too much outside your normal range, it can throw your brain off balance. Prioritise protein at breakfast. Eat more fibre (see page 44). Choose carbohydrates with a low glycaemic index and monitor your overall carbohydrate intake (page 50). Focus on your portion sizes. Although the research is inconclusive, some foods, such as cinnamon, fenugreek seeds and apple cider vinegar, are believed to help lower blood sugars. Don't go crazy with them but they are easy additions to your diet that may help.

GET ENOUGH CHOLINE
Observational studies link choline intake to improved brain function, including better memory and focus. The best sources of choline are liver, fresh cod and eggs. See page 126 for recipe inspiration.

DON'T FEAR FATS
Sixty per cent of your brain is made of fat. Healthy fats like extra virgin olive oil, avocado, nuts and seeds are good additions to your diet. Use extra virgin olive oil daily. Have a closed handful of unsalted, unroasted nuts every day. Keep a mixed seed jar to sprinkle over porridges, salads or soups.

GET COLOURFUL
Phytochemicals, which give the colours to fruit and vegetables, help protect the brain from oxidative stress and also offer memory-boosting agents.

SWAP MILK CHOCOLATE FOR DARK
Dark chocolate (more than 70 per cent cocoa) has antioxidants to boost brain power and mood. The flavonoids also help protect the brain. Chocolate contains some caffeine, which, in small doses, can help with concentration.

TRY GREEN TEA
Green tea is a fantastic alternative to coffee that contains much less caffeine and also contains the L-theanine amino acids, which keep you focused.

SNACK ON A BANANA
Studies show eating bananas helps enhance memory. They contain potassium and vitamin B6, which promotes the production of serotonin and dopamine for concentration. Pair it with walnuts or almonds.

SPICE IT UP

Herbs and spices are packed with antioxidants and nutrients. Incorporating some into your diet every day can promote a healthy brain and reduce inflammation. Add cinnamon to your porridge or pancakes. Mix fresh herbs into salads and soups.

BECOME A FISH FAN

Omega-3s play a role in sharpening memory and improving mood. Eat fish and ensure one portion per week is oily. If you aren't a fish fan, consider taking an omega-3 supplement. Add ground flaxseeds to yoghurt and porridge. Sprinkle pumpkin seeds over salads and soups. Snack on seaweed.

Let's talk about sex

Sex is a taboo subject. Yet sex is good for you! It's an important part of our health and wellbeing. More than half of women say the menopause affects their sex life. Hormonal changes can cause a double whammy – physical changes to your vagina and a loss of interest in sex. I'm no sex expert, so I've presented you with some questions to ask yourself. Based on the responses, you can look at page 255 if you need more support.

> **What is your biggest pain point in terms of vaginal health?** Vaginal dryness, urinary tract infections or pain during sex? Log your symptoms on page 250.
> **How would you rate your level of self-confidence on a scale of one to ten?** One being the lowest and ten being the highest. If your level is below seven, how can you love yourself a little more this week?

What's one thing you can do for yourself to make you feel good?
> **What is your reason for a low sex drive?** Are the physical changes to your vaginal area making sex uncomfortable or painful? Is it your low mood? Are you feeling too tired? Are you stressed or anxious? What is your relationship with your partner like? Is your lifestyle (smoking, alcohol intake or diet) affecting your libido?
> **Are you doing pelvic floor exercises?** Do you know what they are? How often do you do them?
> **Who will you talk about your struggles with?** Are you comfortable talking to your partner about how you feel? Have you spoken to your doctor about your symptoms? Would you benefit from therapy, as an individual or a couple? Do you have any family members or friends you can begin to talk to? Start small.

The research on the link between nutrition and lifestyle and sex is limited, however there are some factors that can have an indirect effect on libido.

GET THE BASICS RIGHT

Eating balanced meals may help your libido. Foods high in protein are also a good source of iron, which is important if fatigue is part of the issue. Limiting your intake of ultra-processed packaged foods can affect your neurotransmitter balance in your brain, which will have a knock-on impact on your mood. Dark green leafy vegetables are packed with magnesium, which helps chill us out.

INCLUDE NATURE'S CARBS

A diet high in sugar, that includes too many processed foods, causes an imbalance in vaginal microbiota. This

More than half of women say the menopause affects their sex life.

leads to vaginal yeast or bacterial infections. Eat more vegetables, berries, legumes, beans and whole grains like barley, and fewer cakes, pastries and sugary drinks.

HYDRATE

Drinking plenty of water helps to ensure the vagina stays well lubricated and helps prevent urinary tract infections. Include cranberry-flavoured herbal teas to increase your fluid intake.

ADD FLAXSEEDS

Healthy fats like olive oil, avocados and flaxseeds can help create a protective mucosal lining inside the vagina. Add a tablespoon of flaxseed to cereal. Add a teaspoon to mustard or hummus. Mix it into muffins and breads.

EAT FERMENTED FOODS

Foods with probiotics, like bio-live yoghurt, kefir, kimchi, sauerkraut, miso and tempeh, help increase the number of good bacteria in the vagina and can help prevent urinary tract infections. Have a shot of kefir every morning. Add sauerkraut or kimchi to your eggs or slip a forkful into salads or sandwiches at lunch. Have a miso soup starter at lunch or dinner. Add tempeh to your stir-fry or bolognese.

BEAT THE BLOAT

Feeling bloated can be a real passion killer. You could look at limiting the amount of gluten you eat. You can also keep a food diary to see which foods make you bloated. Remember, if you're cutting out whole food groups for a long period of time, it's best to speak to a registered nutritional professional.

KEEP ON TOP OF YOUR VITAMIN D LEVELS

Inadequate levels of certain nutrients, such as vitamin D, have been linked with lower sex drive. Vitamin D is crucial in hormone production and sexual health. Get your levels checked and supplement if you need to.

MOVE MORE

Exercise is one of the best ways to bust stress, which is a major libido killer. Good blood flow is necessary for sexual arousal and regular exercise can help with this.

SCHEDULE SOME 'ME TIME'

Invest in yourself by doing some activities that bring you joy. Spend time in sunshine. Soak in a bath. Get your hair done. Put on that red lipstick. Wear that sexy lingerie. Move your body. Quieten your mind and meditate. Phone someone who makes you feel good. Relax in the garden or nature. Go to the cinema. Visit an art gallery. Find your way to get your mojo back.

TAKE IT TO LADIES' NIGHT

Start talking about it. It may be with your close girlfriends or a healthcare professional. Don't suffer in silence.

How to sleep soundly

A recent survey shows 84 per cent of women in the menopause struggle with sleep. Prioritising sleep is always important, even more so during the menopause when the body is more primed to feel the negative effects of stress. I've written about the importance of sleep and given some practical tips already from page 81. However, if you're concerned about your sleep, I invite you to begin to reflect and understand why.

Keeping a sleep diary will give you some insight into your sleep habits. Then begin to ask yourself some key questions: are you struggling to fall asleep or do you wake up in the middle of the night? Are you sleeping seven to nine hours each night? If not, why not? Get to the root of the problem, then you can implement a strategy that will benefit your sleep and your hormones.

DON'T GO LOW CARB

The relationship between diet and sleep is complex. However, some research shows a lack of starchy carbohydrates in your diet means your body is starved of tryptophan, which allows your body to produce melatonin, the sleep hormone. The quality of your carbs matters. Focus on vegetables, whole grains, beans and lentils instead of white rice and bread.

WATCH STIMULANTS

Research suggests that cutting back on nicotine, alcohol and caffeine at least four hours before bed will help with sleep. Making lunch your biggest meal and dinner lighter can also help. If dinner is your biggest meal, try a 15-minute walk after to help with digestion.

PRACTISE THE 3:2:1 RULE

Try three hours of no food, two hours of no work, one hour of no devices. Try reading, listening to music or writing in a journal.

SUPPLEMENT WITH MAGNESIUM

Some sleep experts believe magnesium helps your body's circadian rhythm by regulating the nervous system and relaxing your muscles. Magnesium bisglycinate is thought to promote healthy sleep cycles, however a combined magnesium supplement or a warm bath with Epsom salt may work too.

EXERCISE

It's a reciprocal relationship. Moderate exercise during the day can help you sleep better. Not getting enough sleep may make exercise harder. Start small. Find the best time of day for your workout routine. Experiment with timing and intensity and find what works for you. There's no need to overdo it.

DEAL WITH STRESS

Fill your days with morning sunlight, fresh air, some joyful play time, plenty of deep breaths and connections with others.

SET UP UNWINDING RITUALS

Successful people swear by their daily routines. They claim the key is structure. Do purposeful relaxation exercises before bed. Keep the bedroom cool. Dim the lights, burn some essential oils. Create little rituals.

PART 4

Recipes for success

Kitchen staples

Here are the items I always have on hand to help make eating balanced meals easier, particularly when I am time poor. Use this to help shape your shopping list; many of the recipes in this book use these staple ingredients.

FOOD GROUP	FOOD ITEM
Vegetables and fruit	**Frozen peas.** Can be added to just about anything, from pasta sauces to curries. **Frozen spinach.** I add a couple of cubes to soups or curries. **Jars of peppers in olive oil.** Adds instant plant variety to a meal. **Tinned tomatoes.** A base for most pasta recipes. **Frozen berries.** I use them to make jam and add them to smoothies, porridge, overnight oats or yoghurt. **Dates.** I add them to hot chocolate and to my baking. **Frozen bananas.** Add to smoothies, or defrost and use in Banana and oat pancakes (recipe page 108).
Protein	**Tinned fish.** Sardines, salmon, mackerel and tuna in olive oil. Use for a toast topping or add to veggies and grains for lunch. **Tinned beans.** Chickpeas, kidney beans and butter beans. Add to salads, make hummus or add to one-pan recipes for a fibre boost. **Dried lentils.** Great for easy soups or dhal with spinach. You can also add to stews or casseroles. **Frozen edamame beans.** I throw them in everything for a protein boost. **Eggs.** The best quick meal ever. Eat on seeded toast or add to salad as a protein source.
Carbohydrates	**Quinoa or ancient grains mix.** Add to salads or serve as a side. **Pre-cooked red rice pouches.** No cooking needed. Just heat and add to a meal. **Rolled oats.** A great option for breakfasts, and a delicious addition to baked desserts. **Oatcakes and rye crackers.** Portable healthy carbs; great to eat with dips or as a substitute for bread. **Seeded bread (in the freezer).** A loaf of bread in the freezer is the best. There's no waste.

FOOD GROUP	FOOD ITEM
Healthy fats	**Ground flaxseed.** Store in the fridge and add to porridge, overnight oats, cookies and even mains. **Pumpkin seeds.** Sprinkle over pretty much everything. **Mixed nuts jar.** Almonds, walnuts, brazil nuts, pistachios – add them all in. **Peanut butter and other nut butters.** Store-cupboard staples to support the nut butter addiction! **Tahini.** Great on toast. You can also add it to dressings or use it to make hummus. **Extra virgin olive oil.** The oil I use for cooking and dressings. Works in baking too.
Other items	**Seventy per cent dark chocolate.** A must to satisfy the sweet cravings when they come. **Ground almonds.** A fantastic addition to porridge or baking to boost protein content. **Green tea or matcha powder.** I make a huge mug in the morning and drink it throughout the day cold. **Honey and maple syrup.** Sources of added sugar, but fine to include as part of balanced meals.

The recipes in this section cater for a wide range of dietary needs. Look for the following symbols on the recipes to indicate:

V = vegetarian
VG = vegan
GF = gluten free
DF = dairy free

Recipes also marked with an 'O' will include an option to make the dish suitable for particular dietary needs.
Note that some ingredients, such as stock and ready-made pastes, may not be gluten free; always check the ingredients list of the product to be sure.

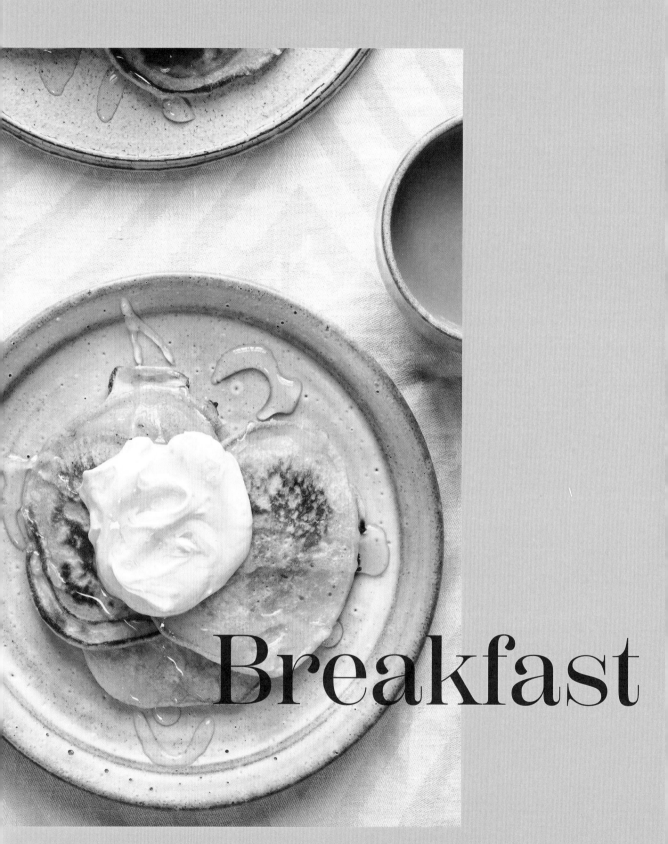

Breakfast

How you begin the morning sets the tone for your day. Make sure you start strong. During the menopause, this means you particularly need to power up the protein. This will help balance your blood-sugar levels, set you up for the rest of the day so you don't get too hungry, and protect your muscle. I find women typically eat a low-protein breakfast, so for all these recipes, I've made protein a big focus, at the same time as making sure they are balanced, hormone-supporting and yummy. They are all quick to put together or can be made the night before. Where milk is featured, you can use your milk of choice; I prefer whole milk and soya.

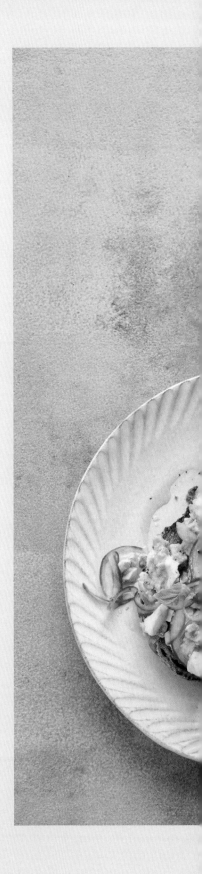

Banana and oat pancakes

Serves 1–2
Ready in 15 minutes

V GF

I love a quick and simple breakfast idea and these banana and oat pancakes are always a hit – kids love them too. They are very easy to make and are so good for your gut. Menopause is linked with a reduced diversity of bacteria in the gut. The more diverse the bacteria, the fewer troublesome symptoms you'll have. Eating a variety of plant-based foods nourishes your bacteria. This recipe is full of all the things that your gut bugs like – and I'm sure you will like them too! They are yum.

1 large ripe banana
50g (½ cup) gluten-free
  rolled oats
1 tbsp ground flaxseed
1 medium egg
1 tbsp peanut butter or nut
  butter of choice
½ tsp baking powder
Splash of milk or plant milk
  of choice, to loosen
Olive oil, to grease the pan
To serve
1 tbsp maple syrup
Large handful of raspberries
Sliced banana

1 Mash the banana with a fork, then transfer to a blender with the oats, flaxseed, egg, peanut butter and baking powder. Whizz together well. Loosen with a little milk to an easily dollopable consistency.

2 Heat a non-stick heavy-based pan over a medium heat and grease lightly with the olive oil. Fry large spoonfuls of the pancake batter for a minute or so on each side until golden brown and puffed.

3 Serve straight away with a drizzle of maple syrup and a scattering of raspberries and sliced banana.

Tip

These freeze, so they're perfect for batch-cooking.

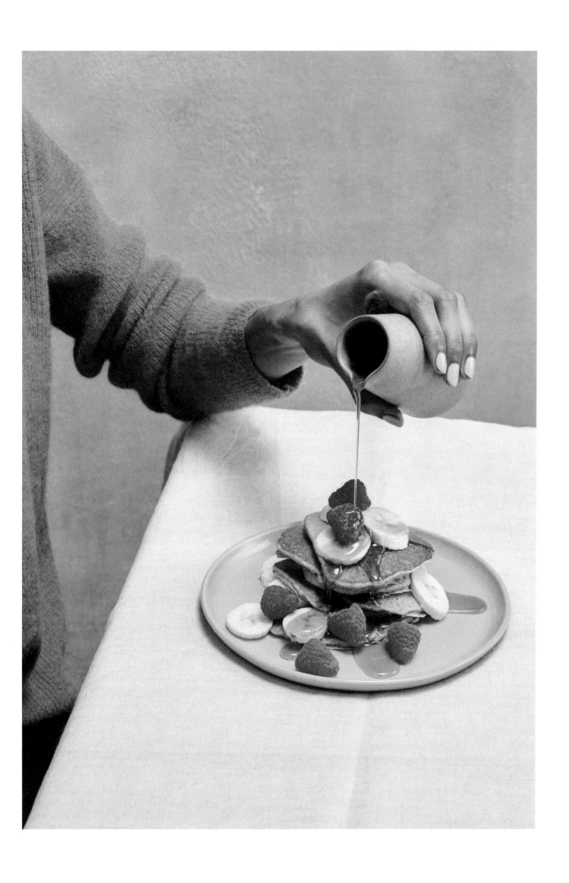

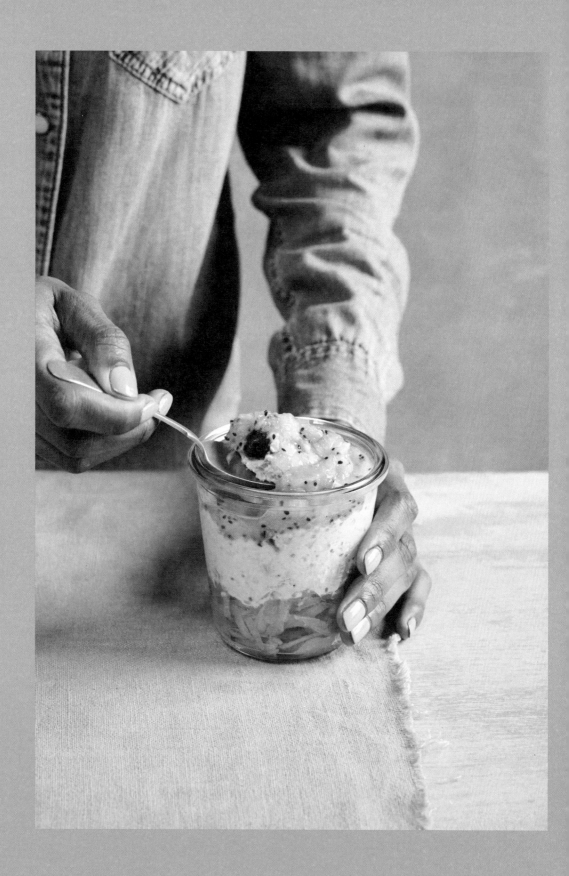

Overnight oats

Makes 4 x 150g (5½oz) jars
Ready in 15 minutes, plus
overnight chilling

V GF

Here is a speedy and versatile alternative to porridge. You can make it the night before and it's also a dish that travels well. It's packed with multiple hero ingredients. Rolled oats are whole grains that release glucose slowly into your blood when digested. Chia seeds are a good source of plant-based omega-3 and a great source of fibre. Kefir is a fermented food that supports a diverse microbiome.

80g (scant 1 cup) gluten-free
  jumbo rolled oats
1 tbsp ground flaxseed
1 tbsp chia seeds
Pinch of ground cinnamon
125g (scant 1 cup) blueberries
200ml (generous ¾ cup) kefir
150ml (generous ½ cup) milk
  or plant milk of choice
3 kiwifruit, peeled
120g (¾ cup) grated carrot

1 Combine the oats, flaxseed, chia seeds and cinnamon in a bowl. Mix in the blueberries, kefir and milk.

2 In a blender, blitz the kiwifruit to a purée.

3 Place the carrot in the bottom of four 150g (5½oz) pots or jars.

4 Spoon the oat mixture on top of the carrot, then top with a layer of kiwi purée.

5 Chill overnight before mixing up and enjoying.

Tip

Try using grated apple instead of carrot, and pomegranate seeds, blended raspberry or blackberry instead of kiwifruit.

High-protein pancakes

Serves 4
Ready in 20 minutes

V

I wanted to create a high-protein pancake recipe that didn't use protein powder. *Voilà*! Protein protects your muscle, and having more muscle boosts your metabolic rate, makes you look more toned, helps keep your body sensitive to insulin and supports strong bones. This recipe uses kefir yoghurt. Kefir is a fermented drink made with milk or water and kefir grains. Kefir yoghurt is a yoghurt that is made with this drink.

125g (scant 1 cup) plain (all-purpose) flour
1 tsp cream of tartar
½ tsp bicarbonate of soda (baking soda)
1 large egg
100g (⅓ cup) cottage cheese
125ml (½ cup) milk or plant milk of choice
1 tsp light olive oil or butter, to grease the pan
To serve
120g (½ cup) Greek yoghurt or thick kefir yoghurt
4 tbsp honey or maple syrup
100g (¾ cup) blueberries (optional)

1 Put the flour, cream of tartar and bicarb in a bowl and mix together. Make a well in the centre, add the egg and cottage cheese, and gradually mix together. Slowly pour in the milk to loosen to a spoonable but not runny consistency.

2 Heat a non-stick heavy-based pan over a medium heat and grease lightly with oil or butter. Fry spoonfuls of the pancake batter for 1–2 minutes each side until golden and puffed up.

3 Serve with dollops of yoghurt, a good drizzle of honey and blueberries, if you like.

Tip

You can try this with silken tofu instead of cottage cheese. Blend it until smooth, then add it to the mixture.

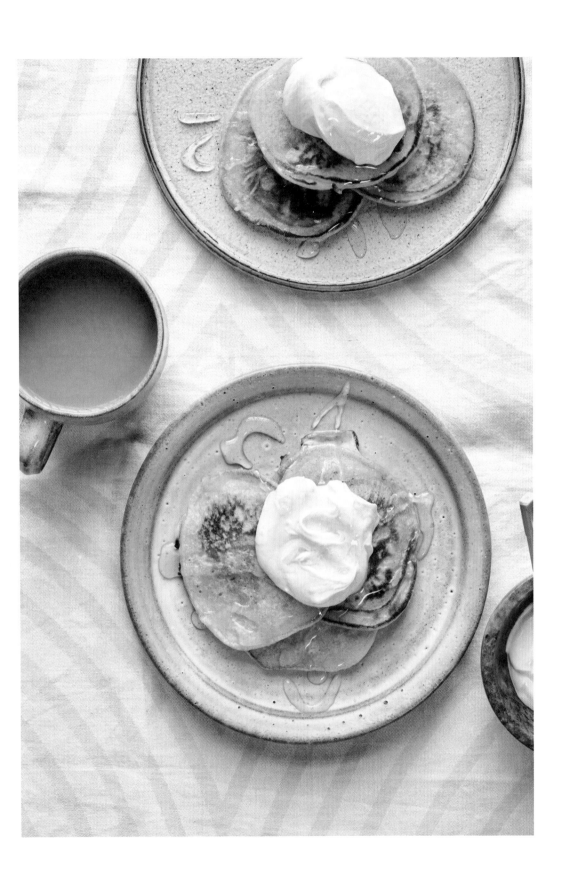

HELPS WITH

No-added-sugar apple and carrot muffins

Makes 12
Ready in 35 minutes, plus cooling time

V GF

While living in Italy, I learned that Italians like to have sweet breakfasts, so I went on a mission to create a sweet start that was also good for me. There is no added sugar here – the sweetness comes from natural sources – and these muffins are perfect for breakfast or an on-the-go afternoon snack. Variety in plant foods and fibre are two things that make your gut bugs thrive. These muffins are bursting with both! Happy gut, healthy you. Women in the menopause need to make feeding their microbes a priority.

1 apple, peeled and cored
    (about 125g/4½oz)
2 carrots, peeled (about
    240g/8½oz)
75g (scant ½ cup) dates, finely
    chopped
60g (½ cup) walnuts, finely
    chopped
200g (2 cups) ground
    almonds
1 heaped tsp baking powder
1 tbsp chia seeds
½ tsp ground cinnamon
1 tsp ground ginger
2 medium eggs
50ml (scant ¼ cup) olive oil
75–100g (¼–⅓ cup) natural
    yoghurt

1 Preheat the oven to 190ºC (375ºF). Line a 12-hole muffin tin with paper cases.

2 Coarsely grate the apple and carrot and put them in a bowl with the dates and walnuts.

3 Add the almond, baking powder, chia seeds, cinnamon and ginger and mix together. In a jug, whisk the egg and oil, add to the bowl and mix well. Add the yoghurt a little at a time until the mixture drops from the spoon.

4 Divide the mixture among the muffin cases and bake for 20-25 minutes until risen and golden and a skewer inserted into the middle comes out clean.

5 Cool in the tin for 10 minutes, then transfer to a wire rack to cool completely.

Tip

These freeze brilliantly, so you can batch-bake and defrost them individually as needed. They will keep in an airtight tin for 2-3 days.

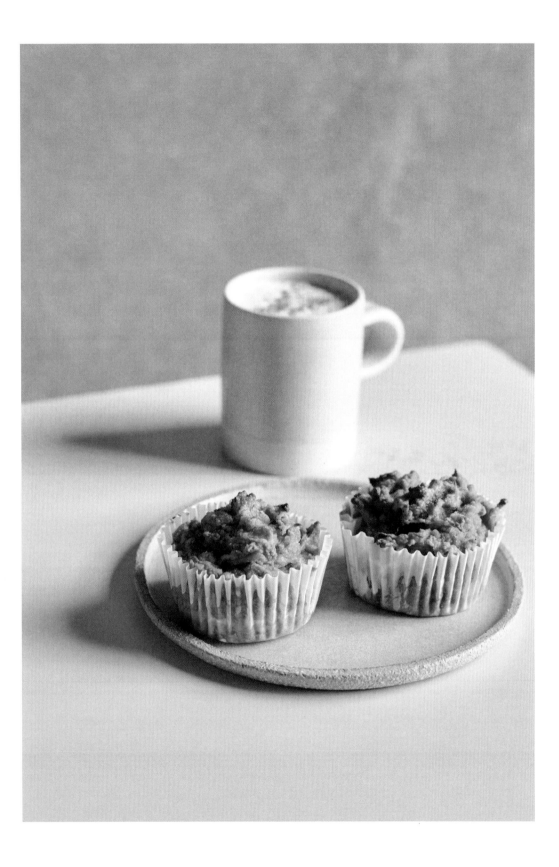

Quinoa porridge

Serves 2
Ready in 15 minutes

VG GF

Many of my clients like to have a porridge as one of their breakfast options. Conventional porridge can be on the low side in terms of protein, making it too carbohydrate-rich. Adding quinoa to this recipe delivers the creamy, comforting feel of porridge but takes it up a notch in protein terms. And quinoa is one of the few plant-based proteins that is a complete protein. Add the soya milk and you also have a good phytoestrogen boost. When I have leftover quinoa, it goes into a porridge. It's a fantastic way to look after yourself and reduce food waste.

100g (3½oz) cooked quinoa
60g (generous ½ cup)
  gluten-free porridge oats
Pinch of sea salt
500ml (2 cups) soya milk,
  plus 100ml (scant
  ½ cup) extra, to serve
4 cardamom pods, cracked,
  or a good pinch of ground
  cardamom
½ tsp ground cinnamon
2 tbsp maple syrup

1 Put the cooked quinoa and porridge oats into a pan with a pinch of salt and the milk, cardamom and cinnamon. Bring to a simmer over a medium heat and cook for 10 minutes, stirring, until the oats are tender. You can loosen with another splash of milk if it starts to thicken too quickly.

2 Spoon into two bowls and top each with a drizzle of maple syrup. Pour over another splash of milk and serve with any toppings you like (see tip).

Tip

Fresh berries, a handful of nuts and seeds, or a dollop of my Blueberry and chia seed jam (see opposite) all make great toppings.

Peanut butter and chia jam on toast

Serves 2 (makes 1 x 370g/13oz jar of jam)
Ready in 20 minutes

VG

2 slices of seeded or
    sourdough bread
2 tbsp smooth or crunchy
    peanut butter, or nut butter
    of choice
1 apple or pear, sliced
Blueberry and chia seed jam
150g (1 cup) blueberries
2 tbsp maple syrup
150ml (generous ½ cup) water
4 tbsp chia seeds

I am a hard-core peanut-butter addict. When I was growing up in Zambia, I probably had peanut butter on toast most days. I would spread the peanut butter as thick as the bread and generously top it with sugar-laden jam. Not very blood-glucose or hormone friendly, right? Thankfully, the dietitian in me has found a version that is much better for my hormones, and just as delicious. The chia seeds are the hero ingredient here, adding some more fibre and a nice little whack of anti-inflammatory omega-3 fats.

1 For the chia jam, put the blueberries, maple syrup and water in a small pan over a medium heat. Bring to a gentle simmer and cook for 10 minutes until the fruit begins to burst. Add the chia seeds and continue to bubble gently for 5–6 minutes until you have a lovely thick, jammy consistency. Allow to cool.

2 Toast your bread, spread with peanut butter and top with your sliced fruit. Spoon over some blueberry and chia jam and serve.

gut health

HELPS WITH

Tip

Leftover chia jam will keep in the fridge in a sterilised jar for a week.

Avo eggs

Serves 2
Ready in 10 minutes

 V DF

2 medium eggs
1 small red onion, finely sliced
Juice of 1 lemon
Pinch of sea salt
1 large ripe avocado
2 slices of seeded or
    sourdough bread
Extra virgin olive oil, to drizzle
Handful of fresh basil leaves
    (optional)

This is one of my favourite go-to breakfast recipes. It's guacamole revisited. I got the inspiration from a good friend of mine, Valentina. She's from South America – the guacamole headquarters! It is scrummy. The avocado is a healthy fat source that will satisfy your tastebuds while nourishing your skin with vitamin E.

1 Put the eggs into a pan of cold water and bring to the boil. Cook for 6 minutes, then drain and cool under cold running water.

2 Meanwhile, put the red onion in a bowl and squeeze over half the lemon. Add a pinch of sea salt and set aside.

3 Roughly mash the avocado in another bowl with the rest of the lemon juice and season with salt and pepper. Peel the eggs, mash with a fork and combine with the avo.

4 Toast the bread, drizzle with a little extra virgin olive oil, then top each slice with half the avo and egg mixture.

5 Add the pretty pink onion and a scattering of basil leaves, along with an extra drizzle of extra virgin olive oil and some freshly ground black pepper.

Tips

I sometimes use apple cider vinegar if I don't have a lemon.
You can boil the eggs in advance – I sometimes even boil my eggs while I shower!

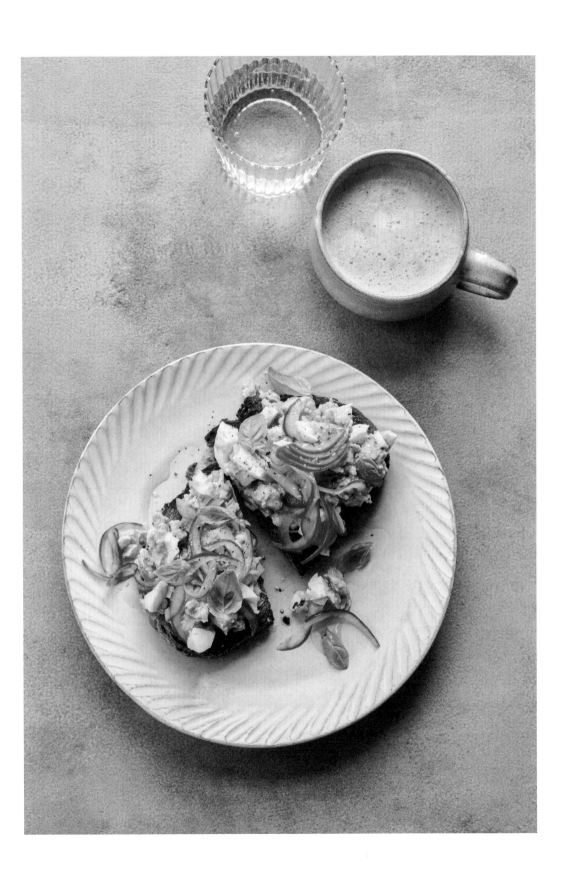

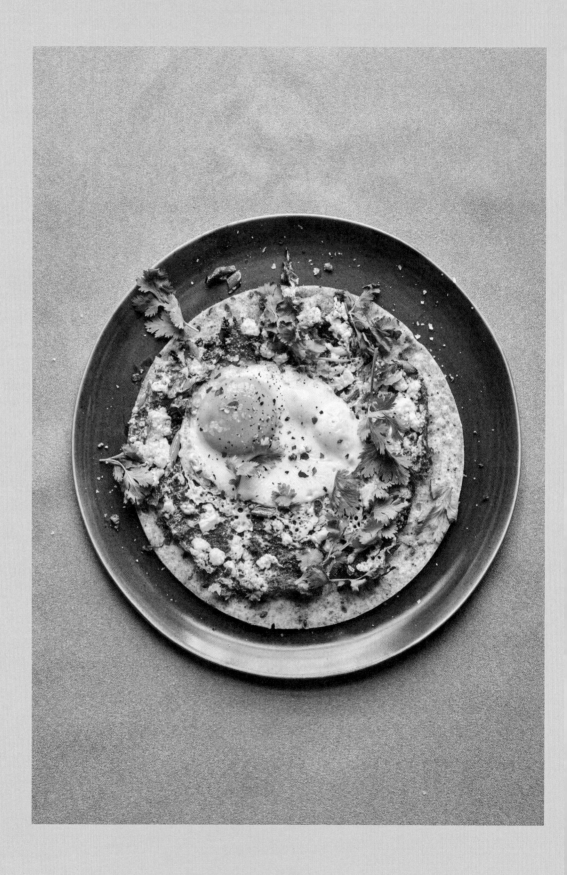

Feta fried eggs

Serves 2
Ready in 20 minutes

This is my take on the feta fried eggs trend that went viral on Instagram in 2023. Eggs are a nutritional powerhouse. They contain 13 different essential vitamins and nutrients, and are one of the greatest sources of choline available. Choline is an essential nutrient that you need to get from foods as your body doesn't produce enough. It's linked with good cognitive function, memory and attention. During the menopause, as your oestrogen levels fall, you are prone to being deficient in choline.

2 tbsp olive oil
1–2 tsp chipotle paste
4 spring onions (scallions), finely sliced
Pinch of sea salt
60g (½ cup) feta cheese, crumbled
2 medium eggs
2 small seeded flour tortillas, warmed
Large handful of fresh coriander (cilantro) leaves (optional)

1 Heat half the oil in a non-stick frying pan over a medium-high heat and fry ½–1 tsp of the chipotle paste and half of the spring onion with a pinch of sea salt for 1–2 minutes until softened.

2 Add half the feta and let it cook, undisturbed, for 2 minutes, then crack one egg on top. Cook for another 2 minutes until the white is slightly crispy and the yolk starts to set, then season with a little sea salt and freshly ground black pepper. Remove, drain briefly on kitchen towel, slide onto a tortilla and garnish with coriander, if using.

3 Repeat with the other half of the ingredients and serve.

Tips

This is delicious served with slices of avocado. You can also try using harissa paste instead of chipotle.

Bang bang beans

Serves 2
Ready in 20 minutes

VG

I love toast for a simple breakfast, but sometimes I have to think outside the box about what I put on top! Experts all over the world agree that perimenopausal and menopausal women should eat more fibre. Fibre not only keeps you fuller for longer, but also feeds your gut bacteria, which are key in regulating your oestrogen levels. Beans are a fantastic source of fibre. What I love about this dish is that you can make it in advance and add whatever extra veggies you have in the fridge to mix it up. Serve with a slice of sourdough toast for breakfast and a baked potato or wrap for lunch.

2 tbsp olive oil
2 sprigs of fresh oregano, leaves stripped, or ½ tsp dried
150g (1¼ cups) cherry tomatoes
100ml (scant ½ cup) water
1 tbsp tomato paste (concentrated purée)
1 x 400g (14oz) tin cannellini beans, drained and rinsed
1 tsp hot smoked paprika
2 tsp soft dark brown sugar
2 tsp apple cider vinegar
2 slices of seeded or sourdough toast, to serve

1 Heat the oil in a pan over a high heat. Add the oregano and cherry tomatoes and cook for 5 minutes until they start to blister and burst. At this point, add the water and the tomato paste, and press down on the tomatoes with your spoon to make a lovely sauce.

2 Add the beans, paprika, sugar and vinegar, and season with sea salt and freshly ground black pepper. Simmer for 12–15 minutes.

3 Serve with seeded or sourdough toast.

Tip

This is a really great dish for a weekend breakfast, but if you fancy it midweek, you can make it even simpler by using 2 tsp chipotle chilli paste rather than the smoked paprika, sugar and vinegar.

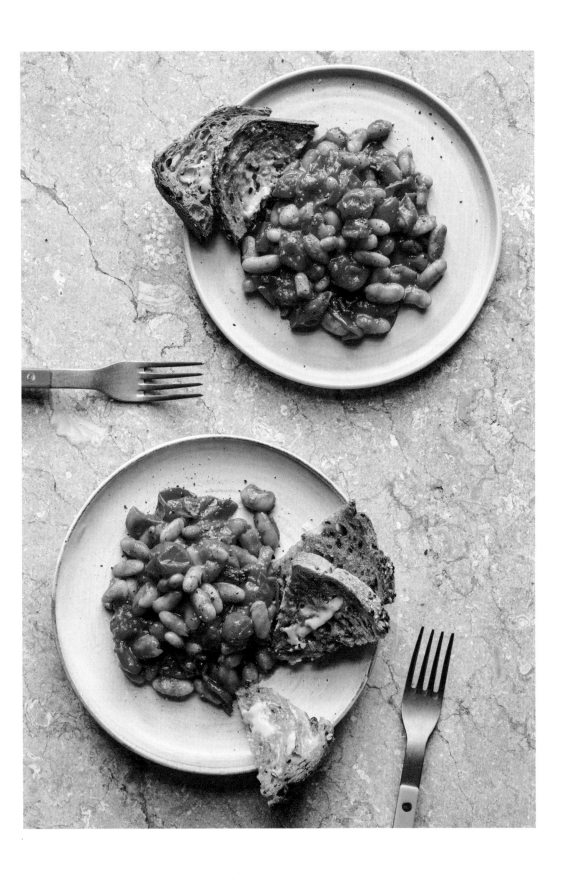

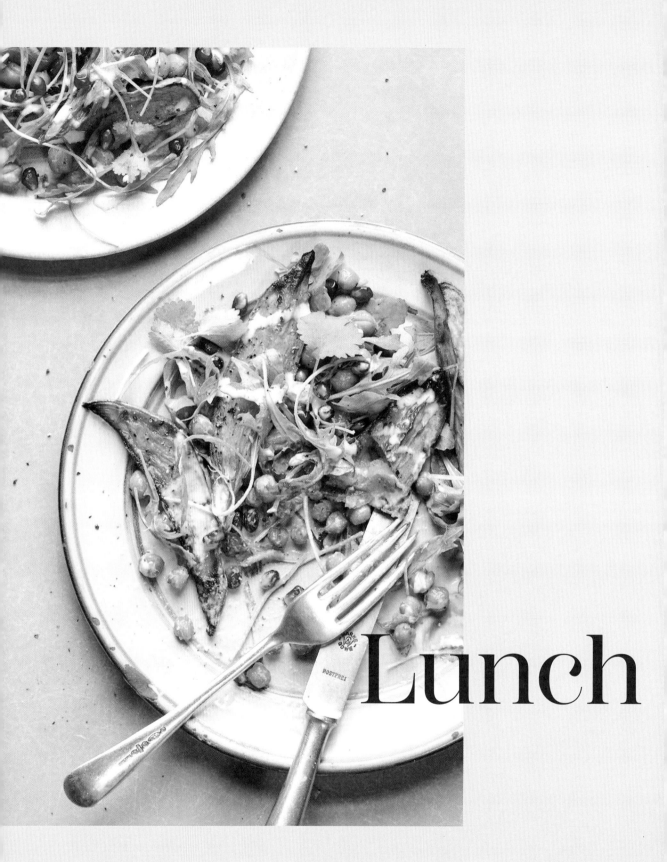

Lunch

Lunchtime fuelling is important. Depending on what you eat, it can energise you or cause you to have an afternoon slump and have you reaching for a biscuit at around 4pm. These weekday lunches are easy to make and perfectly balanced, with lots of colourful veggies, lean protein, slow-release carbs and healthy fats to ensure you're well nourished for a productive afternoon.

Research shows that during menopause, women can become sensitive, or more sensitive, to salt, so it can have a bigger impact on your health than it did previously. I have not stipulated the salt intake in these recipes, so you can season as you desire, but I would recommend going easy on the salt.

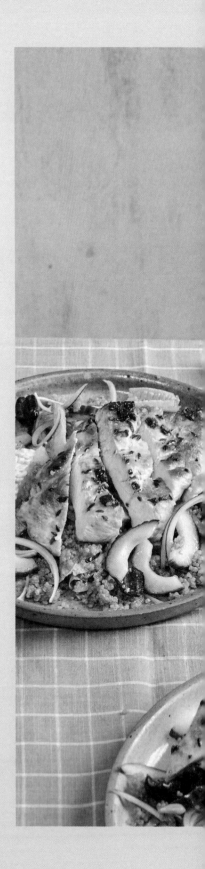

Frittata

Serves 4–6
Ready in 45 minutes

V GF

Nutritionally, frittatas can be fantastic, as they provide you with good protein and you can add all sorts of plant-based goodness to them. But I find a lot of frittatas a bit dry and bland. Not this one, baby! I have packed in the nutrition and the taste. The broad beans are my star ingredient here. You have heard me say it before, and I will keep saying it – we need to eat more fibre! Beans are a brilliant source of fibre. Broad beans are also bursting with folate, which new research suggests could help support hot flushes.

2 courgettes (zucchini) (about 350g/12oz), coarsely grated
Pinch of sea salt
2 tbsp olive oil
4 spring onions (scallions), finely sliced
6 medium eggs
2 tbsp finely chopped fresh dill
Finely grated zest of 1 lemon
75g (¾ cup) grated vegetarian hard cheese or parmesan
200g (1⅓ cups) frozen broad beans, defrosted

1 Put the courgette into a sieve and sprinkle with a good pinch of sea salt. Allow to sit for 10 minutes, then squeeze out as much liquid as possible.

2 Heat the grill to medium-high.

3 Heat the olive oil in a 20cm (8-inch) ovenproof non-stick frying pan over a medium-high heat. Add the spring onion and courgette and fry for 3–4 minutes.

4 Meanwhile, in a jug, use a stick blender to blend the egg with the dill, lemon zest and cheese. Season to taste with salt and black pepper.

5 Add the broad beans to the frying pan, then pour over the egg mixture and stir well.

6 Reduce the heat to medium-low and cook for 4–5 minutes until the frittata is set about two-thirds of the way through. Pop under the grill for 5-6 minutes until golden and puffy, then leave to sit for 10 minutes in the pan before loosening with a spatula. Slide onto a serving board or plate to serve.

Tip

You could swap the broad beans for peas or edamame.

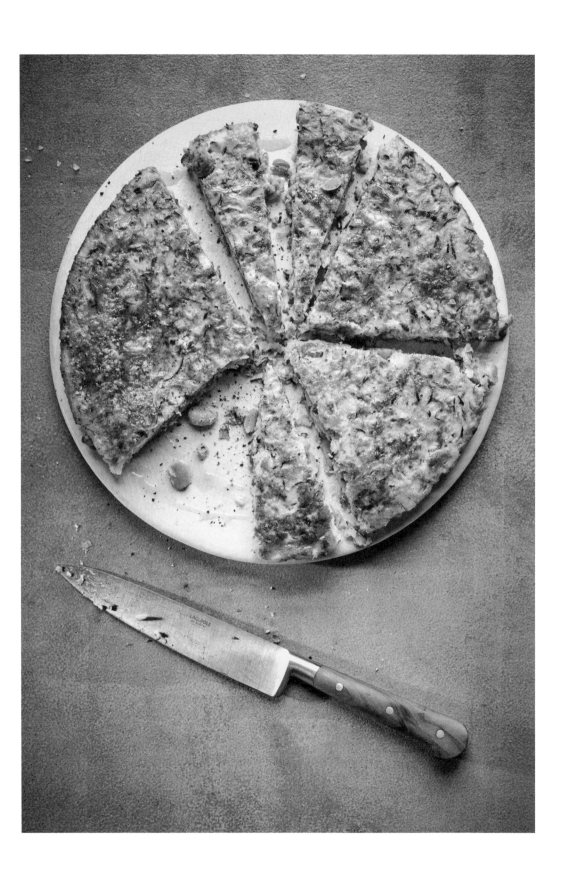

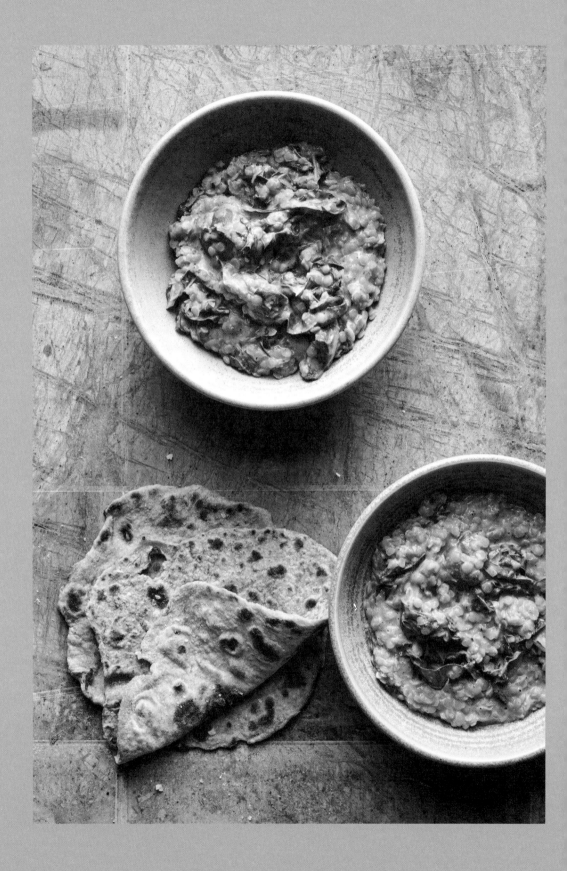

Red lentil dhal with spinach and homemade sweet potato chapatis

Serves 4–6
Ready in 1 hour

V

1 tbsp olive oil
1 red onion, finely chopped
2 cloves garlic, whole
   (optional)
3cm (1¼ inch) piece of fresh
   ginger, peeled and grated
1 tbsp garam masala
1 tsp ground turmeric
350g (1⅔ cups) red split lentils
150g (5½oz) tomatoes,
   chopped
1 x 400ml (14fl oz) tin coconut
   milk
300ml (1¼ cups) fresh
   vegetable stock (or use a
   low-sodium stock cube)
100g (⅔ cup) plain
   (all-purpose) flour

Sweet potato chapatis
1 sweet potato (about
   200g/7oz)
150g (1¼ cups) wholemeal
   chapati flour (or wholemeal
   flour whizzed in the food
   processor and sieved)
Pinch of salt
1 tsp ground cumin
3 tbsp kefir yoghurt or natural
   yoghurt
200g (7oz) baby spinach

When I was growing up, my mum had a fusion Indian-Zambian restaurant, and dhal was one of the first recipes she taught me to cook. It's comforting and a real crowd-pleaser – and the sweet-potato chapatis are wow. This also gets gold stars in terms of nutrition for happy hormones. Lentils are rich in protein, fibre and B vitamins, which are essential for mood regulation. Vitamin B6 also serves as a co-factor for enzymes involved with oestrogen metabolism.

1 Preheat the oven to 200°C (400°F). Roast the sweet potato for the chapatis for 40 minutes until tender.

2 Meanwhile, to make the dhal, heat the oil in a pan over a medium heat and fry the onion for 10 minutes until softened. Add the garlic, if using, along with the ginger, garam masala and turmeric and fry for a minute more. Add the lentils, tomato, coconut milk and stock. Season and simmer for 15 minutes until the liquid has been absorbed and the dhal has thickened.

3 To make the chapatis, when cool enough to handle, scoop out the sweet potato flesh from its skin and mash in a bowl. Add the flours, a good pinch of salt and the cumin and yoghurt. Bring together into a dough and divide into six portions. Roll out each portion to a few millimetres thick. Heat a heavy-based frying pan over a medium heat and dry-fry the breads, in batches, for 3–4 minutes on both sides until they are cooked and golden.

4 Meanwhile, add the spinach to the dhal and allow it to wilt. Remove the garlic cloves, if using, and discard. Serve the dhal with the chapatis.

Tips

Roast the sweet potato ahead of time and keep the mashed flesh in the fridge for up to a week.
If you're short on time, you can serve the dhal with bought flatbreads or chapatis.
This recipe is good for batch-cooking and freezing.

Healthy summer rolls
with dipping sauce

Serves 4
Ready in 40 minutes

DF GF

When I remember to make these, I always become obsessed with them for a period of time, as they are so good. They are a great way to make tofu taste delicious, but you can fill them with your protein of choice – roast chicken or even prawns. Sometimes I use smoked instead of plain tofu. Tofu and soy-rich foods are a source of phytoestrogens, which are compounds similar to human oestrogen. Including tofu in your diet can help to soften some of the effects of falling oestrogen. Please note these effects are much weaker than HRT, so if you're taking HRT, you need to keep taking it! If you feel you may have gluten sensitivity, this dish is also for you.

1 tbsp sesame oil
280g (10oz) block firm tofu,
   cut into flat batons
2 tsp gluten-free soy sauce
1 tsp honey
Pinch of chilli flakes
8 rice paper wraps or large
   iceberg lettuce leaves
1 carrot, cut into matchsticks
½ cucumber, deseeded and
   cut into matchsticks
1 ripe avocado, finely sliced
Large handful of fresh
   coriander (cilantro) leaves
   (optional)
Handful of fresh mint leaves
Dipping sauce
1 tbsp rice vinegar
Juice of 1 lime
1 small green chilli, finely
   sliced
1 tbsp gluten-free fish sauce
1 tsp caster (superfine) sugar

1 Heat the sesame oil in a large non-stick frying pan over a medium-high heat and fry the tofu for 4–5 minutes until golden and crisp on all sides. Add the soy sauce, honey and chilli flakes, and cook for a further minute or two until lovely and sticky. Set aside.

2 Whisk together all the ingredients for the dipping sauce in a bowl.

3 To assemble the rolls, dip a rice paper wrap into a bowl of water until it begins to soften, then lay on a chopping board. (If you're using lettuce leaves instead, there is no need to soak them.) Top with some of the tofu, carrot, cucumber and avocado, as well as some herbs. Fold in the sides and then roll into a sausage shape. Repeat with the remaining wraps and filling.

4 Serve the rolls with the dipping sauce.

Tips

Try dipping your tofu in sesame seeds before frying, or putting a piece of nori on top of your rice paper wrap before rolling. You could also add a sprinkle of sesame seeds to the filling.
You can just use soy sauce instead of the dipping sauce.

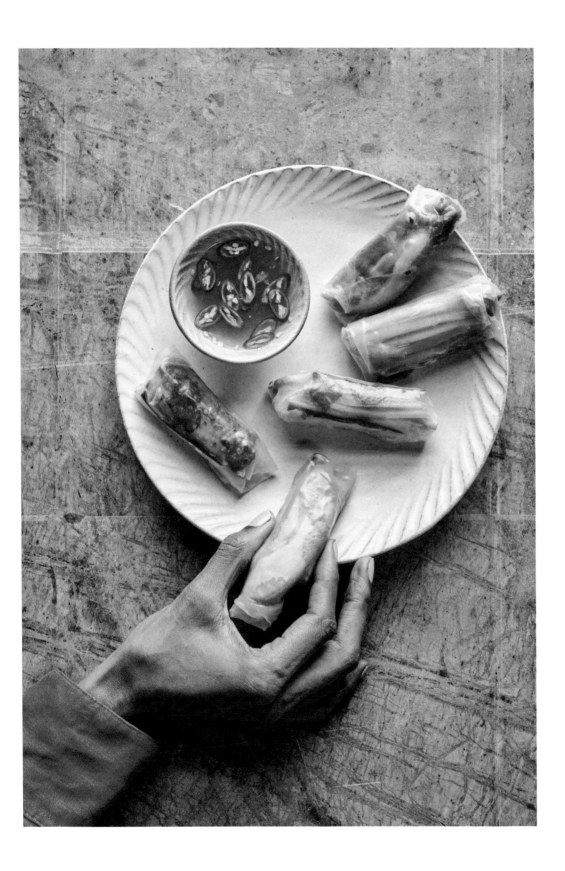

Easy broccoli pesto pasta

Serves 4
Ready in 20 minutes

Since I've been living in Italy, pasta has become a staple. Rather than making creamy sauces, you can begin to use more veggies in your pasta. I love this recipe, as it takes pesto to another level in terms of both taste and nutrition. Broccoli and other cruciferous veggies are star additions to your diet as they contain a chemical called indole-3 carbinol, which supports the liver to work more efficiently, helping to counter the effects of high oestrogen-progesterone, for example. This recipe needs a protein side to round it out, so serve with an extra handful of edamame beans and give yourself a pat on the back for balancing things so well.

450g (1lb) rigatoni or other short pasta
½ head of broccoli, cut into florets
30g (1oz) pine nuts or blanched hazelnuts, toasted
Handful of fresh flat-leaf parsley, leaves picked
Handful of fresh basil, leaves picked
1 fat clove garlic, crushed (optional)
30g (⅓ cup) grated pecorino cheese
Juice of ½ lemon
3–4 tbsp extra virgin olive oil or Garlic oil (see page 224)
Grated pecorino cheese, extra, to serve (optional)

1 Bring a large pan of salted water to the boil. Add the pasta and cook for 10 minutes until al dente.

2 Meanwhile, steam or blanch the broccoli for 2–3 minutes until tender, then cool under cold running water.

3 Place the broccoli in a food processor. Add the nuts, herbs and garlic, if using, along with the cheese. Blitz together, then add the lemon juice and drizzle in the extra virgin olive oil until you have a lovely rich pesto, seasoning with salt and pepper to taste.

4 Drain the pasta, reserving a small cup of the cooking water. Toss the pasta with the pesto, adding a little cooking water to loosen it. Serve with extra cheese, if you like.

Tips

Any leftover pesto will keep in the fridge for up to a week. Be sure to cook the pasta al dente as this keeps the glycaemic index low.

Crispy mushroom and black bean quesadillas

Serves 4
Ready in 35 minutes

V

I love a quesadilla, and this one keeps your fat portions in check too! This recipe is meant to be versatile, so you can include all sorts of extras, from chicken, tofu or Quorn to whatever veggies you have in the fridge/freezer. The one ingredient that is a must is the mushrooms. Mushrooms are so packed with health benefits they are almost medicinal. They contain immune-modulating nutrients, plus beta-glucan, a type of soluble fibre that benefits your gut bacteria.

3 tbsp olive oil
300g (10½oz) mushrooms, sliced
1 red onion, finely sliced
1 tsp chipotle paste
1 x 400g (14oz) tin black beans, drained and rinsed
Large handful of fresh coriander (cilantro), chopped (optional)
4 tortilla wraps (see page 226 for recipe or shop-bought)
120g (1¼ cups) grated cheese (Wensleydale, cheddar, mozzarella)
8 tbsp kefir or natural yoghurt, to serve
2 ripe avocados, sliced, to serve (optional)

1 Heat half the olive oil in a frying pan over a high heat and fry the mushroom for 4–5 minutes, stirring occasionally, until golden and crisp.

2 Add the onion and fry for a further 4–5 minutes, then add the chipotle and black beans. Cook for 2–3 minutes more, then remove from the heat and stir in the coriander, if using.

3 Heat half the oil in a clean non-stick pan over a medium-high heat and add a tortilla. Top with half of the mushroom mixture and half the cheese, then add a second tortilla on top. Fry for 2 minutes, then flip over and fry for 2 minutes more until golden and melty.

4 Slide onto a board and repeat with the remaining ingredients. Slice the quesadillas into wedges and serve with yoghurt and slices of avocado, if using.

gut health

HELPS WITH

Tip

You can serve this with a quick tomato salsa. Finely chop 120g (¾ cup) cherry tomatoes and toss with a little finely chopped red onion, some defrosted frozen sweetcorn, chilli flakes, lime juice and some extra virgin olive oil.

Crispy kimchi and tofu buddha bowls

Serves 2
Ready in 40 minutes

DF GF

YUMMY! This recipe may look a bit of a faff to make, but it honestly isn't. It's a balanced bowl, bursting with flavour and goodness. The kimchi is your hero ingredient here as it's your something fermented for the day. Fermented foods like kimchi or sauerkraut are incredible probiotics (live bacteria), working in unison with your own gut microbiota to create a thriving ecosystem in your intestines. Ideally, you should be eating something fermented every day for optimal gut health.

120g (⅔ cup) wild rice
  or red rice
1 tbsp Garlic oil (see
  page 224)
200g (7oz) firm tofu, cut into
  cubes and patted dry
3cm (1¼ inch) piece of fresh
  ginger, cut into matchsticks
150g (5½oz) curly kale,
  shredded
150g (5½oz) kimchi
2 tsp sesame seeds, toasted
Sauce
2 tsp sesame oil
3 tbsp gluten-free soy sauce
2 tbsp rice vinegar
2 tsp honey

1 Cook the rice in a saucepan of salted boiling water according to the packet instructions until just tender, then drain. Return to the pan, cover with a lid and leave to steam dry.

2 Meanwhile, to make the sauce, whisk together all the ingredients in a small bowl and set aside.

3 Heat the garlic oil in a frying pan over a medium-high heat and fry the tofu and ginger for 5 minutes until crispy and golden on all sides. Scoop out onto a plate lined with kitchen towel to drain.

4 Steam the kale for 2–3 minutes until tender.

5 Divide the rice among four bowls. Top with the kale, tofu and kimchi and drizzle with the sauce. Scatter with sesame seeds and serve.

Tips

Instead of kale, try broccoli, asparagus, green beans or king oyster mushrooms. To save time, you can use a pouch of cooked wild rice.

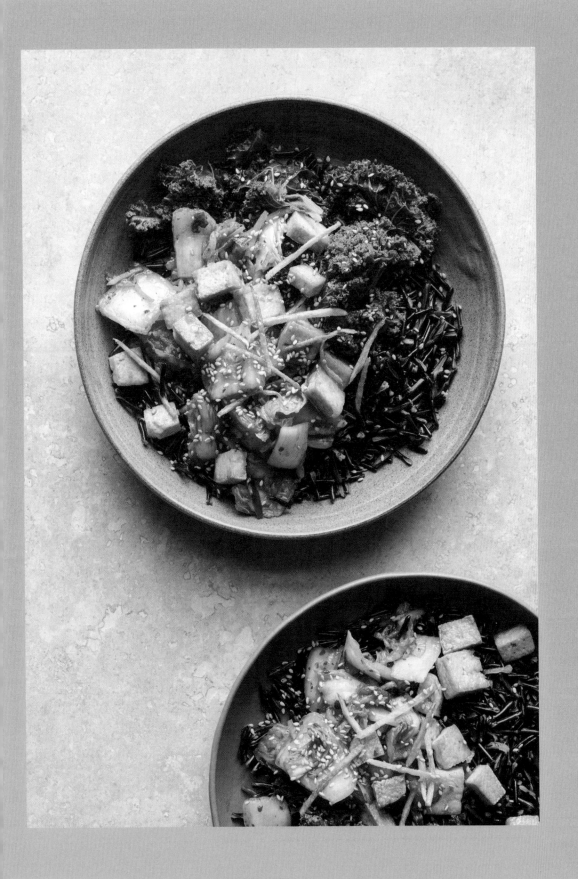

Greek chicken and quinoa salad

Serves 2
Ready in 20 minutes

DF GF

Salads don't have to just be green leaves! This is kinda like a Greek salad, but it's been majorly pimped to help balance your hormones. Bursting with plant points, it's a winner for your gut microbiota. It also contains red onion, which I'm a big fan of. Red onions are an excellent source of antioxidants and contain at least 17 types of flavonoids – key for reducing the oxidative stress our cells experience as part of aging. If you feel you may have gluten sensitivity, this one is for you.

2 small chicken breasts
2 sprigs of fresh oregano,
  leaves stripped, or 1 tsp dried
½ tsp cumin seeds
1 tbsp olive oil
120g (4¼oz) cooked quinoa
1 romaine lettuce, choppped
⅓ cucumber, deseeded and
  sliced into half-moons
½ red onion, finely sliced
10 black olives
Dressing
Juice of ½ lemon
Pinch of cayenne pepper
2 tbsp extra virgin olive oil

1 Flatten the chicken breasts between two pieces of parchment paper. Season with sea salt and freshly ground black pepper, then scatter over the oregano and cumin seeds.

2 Heat the oil in a non-stick frying pan over a medium-high heat and fry the chicken for 3–4 minutes each side or until golden and cooked through. Remove from the pan and leave to cool, then slice into strips.

3 Divide the quinoa between two plates. Toss the lettuce, cucumber and onion together in a bowl and divide between the plates, then top with the chicken and scatter with the olives.

4 To make the dressing, whisk the lemon juice in a small bowl with some salt and pepper and cayenne pepper, then gradually whisk in the oil. Pour over the salad and serve.

Tips

Cook the chicken in advance (or use leftover roast chicken) to make things easier.
You can use wild rice or buckwheat instead of quinoa, and add pumpkin seeds (pepitas) for extra crunch.

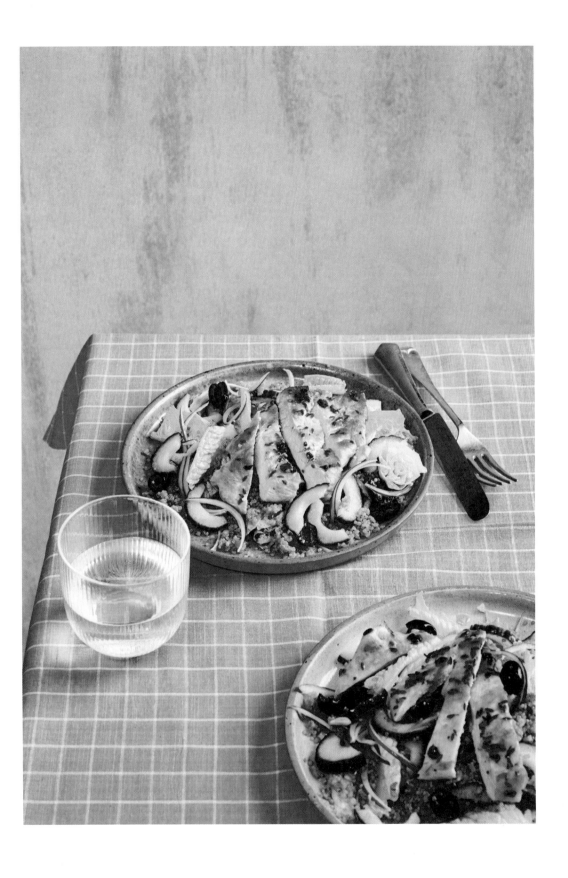

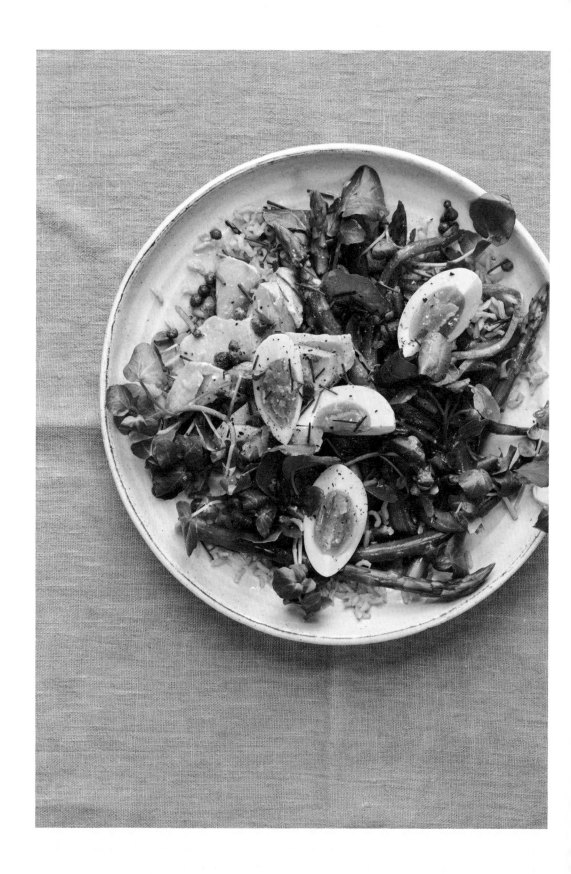

Salmon niçoise

Serves 2
Ready in 15 minutes

DF GF

This is the anti-inflammatory salad of your dreams. Salmon is rich in protein and contains anti-inflammatory omega-3 fats. Wild rice is a fantastic gluten-free, slow-release carbohydrate. Watercress is a cruciferous vegetable that is a great source of beta-carotene, vitamin E, vitamin C and two powerful antioxidants – lutein and zeaxanthin. All these nutrients also work together to keep levels of inflammation low as they lap up free radicals, which can cause damage as we age.

120g (⅔ cup) quick-cook rice (or 250g cooked wild or brown rice from a microwave pouch)
2 medium eggs
150g (5½oz) French green beans
10 asparagus spears
100g (3½oz) watercress
2 poached salmon fillets, flaked
1 tbsp capers
25g (1oz) fresh chives, snipped

Dressing
Juice of ½ lemon
1 tsp Dijon mustard
1 tsp honey
2 tbsp extra virgin olive oil

1 Cook the rice in a saucepan of salted boiling water according to the packet instructions until just tender, then drain. Return to the pan, cover and leave to steam dry.

2 Meanwhile, put the eggs into a pan of cold water. Bring to the boil and boil for 6 minutes, then drain and run under cold water to cool completely.

3 Bring another pan of water to the boil and blanch the beans and asparagus for 2–3 minutes, then drain and refresh under cold water to stop the cooking.

4 Divide the wild rice, watercress, beans and asparagus between two plates and scatter over the salmon. Peel the eggs, cut into quarters and arrange on top.

5 For the dressing, whisk the lemon juice with the Dijon mustard, honey and salt and pepper, then whisk in the extra virgin olive oil.

6 Scatter the capers over the salad, drizzle with the dressing and top with the chives and some freshly ground black pepper.

Tips

For a winter version, swap the beans and asparagus for finely shredded raw brussels sprouts or red cabbage. You could also swap the salmon for sardines in olive oil or mackerel.
You can cook the wild rice ahead of time; cool it quickly by spreading it out on a tray, then keep it in the fridge for up to 5 days.

Roasted sweet potato and chickpea salad with pomegranate

Serves 2
Ready in 1 hour

V GF

This is me wanting to be Yotam Ottolenghi! It's a delicious plant-based recipe that gives you 23 grams of protein per serve. Sweet potatoes fall into the healthy starchy carb category – they are high in fibre and low on the glycaemic index. They are also rich in immune-supporting vitamins and contain three antioxidants: beta-carotene, chlorogenic acid and anthocyanins, which all help reduce the level of oxidative stress in our bodies. Your skin will thank you.

2 medium sweet potatoes (about 375g/13oz), cut into wedges
2 tbsp Garlic oil (see page 224)
1 x 400g (14oz) tin chickpeas, drained and rinsed
1 tsp ground cumin
1 tsp ground coriander
Good pinch of cayenne pepper
100g (3½oz) rocket (arugula) leaves
Large handful of fresh coriander (cilantro), chopped (optional)
Seeds from ½ pomegranate
Dressing
Juice of ½ lemon
2 tsp tahini
1 tbsp natural yoghurt
2 tbsp extra virgin olive oil

1 Preheat the oven to 200ºC (400ºF).

2 Arrange the sweet potato wedges on a roasting tray and drizzle with the garlic oil. Season with sea salt and freshly ground black pepper and roast for 30–35 minutes, turning once, until tender and golden.

3 Add the chickpeas and spices, toss together, and roast for a further 10 minutes.

4 For the dressing, whisk the lemon juice with the tahini and a little salt and pepper, then whisk in the natural yoghurt and extra virgin olive oil. Loosen with a splash of cold water.

5 Divide the sweet potato and chickpeas betwween two plates and top with the rocket leaves and coriander, if using. Scatter with the pomegranate seeds and serve drizzled with the dressing.

Tips

You can roast the sweet potato and chickpeas a day or two in advance and just heat through while you make the dressing.
You can swap out the chickpeas for any beans you like. I love adding edamame beans.

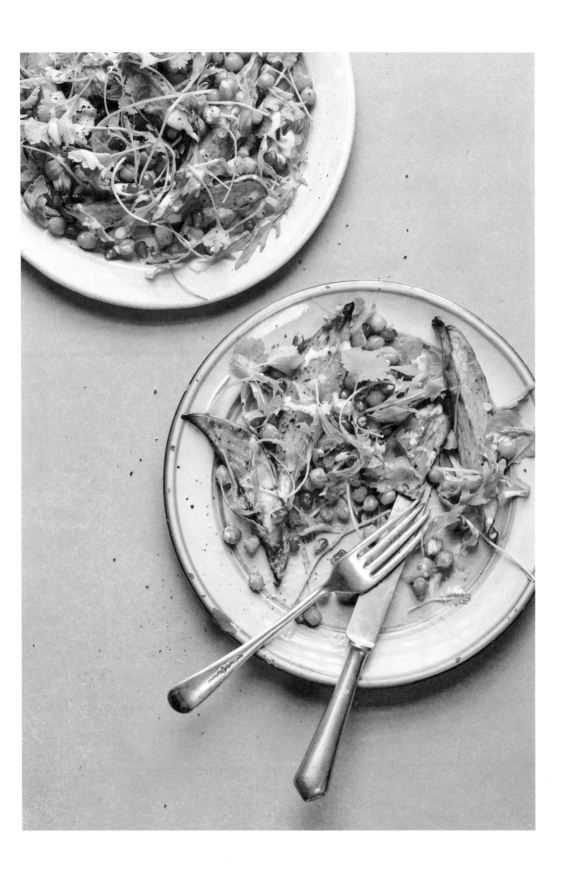

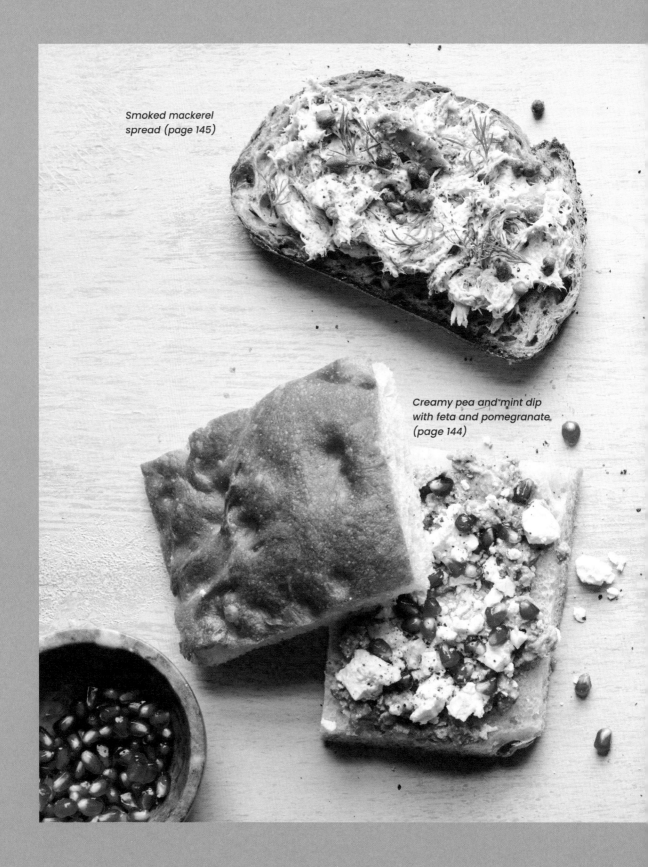

Smoked mackerel
spread (page 145)

Creamy pea and mint dip
with feta and pomegranate
(page 144)

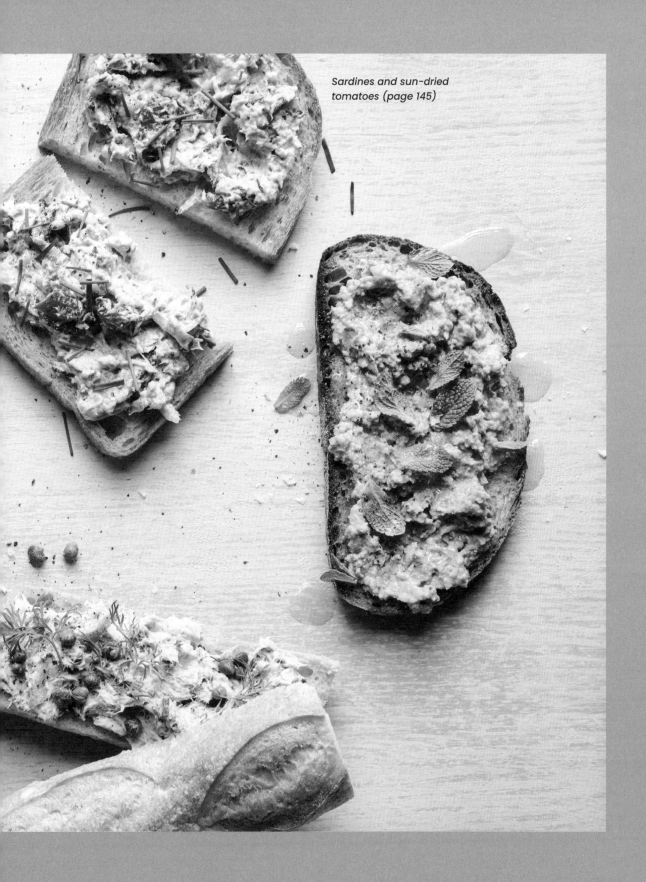

Sardines and sun-dried tomatoes (page 145)

Open sandwiches

Something-on-toast lunches – the best thing since sliced bread! Coming up with quick and healthy lunches can be a challenge. Classic sandwiches are often the best choices for our hormones. Here are some ways I have made my 'something-on-toast' lunches nutritious, filling and, of course, delicious. You can make them gluten free by using gluten-free bread.

Creamy pea and mint dip with feta and pomegranate

Makes 4 open sandwiches
Ready in 20 minutes

V

200g (scant 1½ cups) frozen peas, defrosted
2 tbsp crème fraiche
Small sprig of fresh mint, leaves finely chopped
4 slices of seeded or sourdough bread, toasted, if you like
60g (½ cup) feta cheese, crumbled
Seeds from ½ pomegranate

This recipe may seem quirky, but it's quick to put together and adaptable. The star ingredient here is the pomegranate seeds. Visually, I think they take any dish up a level. Taste-wise, they add a nice refreshing touch. Nutritionally, pomegranates are also a powerful addition. They contain a substance called urolithin A. New research suggests that this boosts the mitochondria – our cells' 'energy power stations'. More energy, anyone?

1 Put the peas into a small food processor. Add the crème fraiche and mint and blend together with some sea salt and black pepper.

2 Spread onto the seeded or sourdough bread or toast slices, scatter with the feta cheese and pomegranate and serve.

Tip

Swap out the peas for edamame beans or broad beans.

Sardines and sun-dried tomatoes

Makes 4 open sandwiches
Ready in 15 minutes

Sardines are a wonderful source of omega-3 fatty acids and they are the most economical omega-3 fish option out there. Not only are they rich in essential fats, they are also a good source of protein and a great source of non-dairy calcium.

1 x 125g (4½oz) tin sardine fillets in olive oil, drained
2 tbsp Greek or natural yoghurt
¼ cucumber, grated and squeezed dry
1 tbsp finely chopped fresh chives
4 sun-dried tomatoes, sliced
4 slices of seeded or sourdough bread

1 Mash the sardines, yoghurt and cucumber together in a bowl and season with salt and pepper to taste. Stir in the chives and sun-dried tomatoes.

2 Toast the bread, then top with the sardines.

Tip

You can also add sliced red onion and rocket or sliced cucumber and basil on top of the sardines.

Smoked mackerel spread

Makes 4 open sandwiches
Ready in 15 minutes

When I'm in back-to-back Zoom meetings with limited time to whip up lunch, this is one of the recipes I fall back on. It uses store-cupboard ingredients, there's no cooking needed and it's delicious. The high protein content can help stabilise blood-sugar levels and keep you feeling satisfied.

150g (5½oz) smoked mackerel
2 tbsp cream cheese
1 tbsp natural yoghurt
1 tbsp capers, chopped
Finely grated zest of 1 lemon and a squeeze of juice
1 tbsp each chopped fresh chives and dill, or 1 tsp dried
4 slices sourdough bread

1 Put the mackerel in a bowl with the cream cheese and yoghurt and mash together, then add the capers, lemon zest and juice and herbs. Serve on sourdough bread.

Tip

This spread will keep in the fridge for 4-5 days.

HELPS WITH: healthy joints | mood regulation | concentration

HELPS WITH: mood regulation | blood-glucose control

Spicy mushrooms and caramelised onion with crispy kale on toast

Makes 2 open sandwiches
Ready in 25 minutes

VG

150g (5½oz) curly kale,
   thick stems removed
2 tbsp olive oil
1 tbsp sesame seeds
1 large red onion, finely sliced
300g (10½oz) king oyster
   mushrooms, shredded
Good pinch of chilli flakes
1 tsp apple cider vinegar
2 tsp gluten-free soy sauce
2 slices of seeded or
   sourdough bread
1 tbsp extra virgin olive oil

This works so well as a light and delish lunch option. It's bursting with plant-based goodness, but the hero ingredient is the mushrooms. Although low in calories, mushrooms pack in plenty of nutrients. They are one of the few plant-based foods that contain some vitamin B12. They also contain vitamin D2 and are higher in protein than most veggies. They contain many bio-active compounds that are thought to improve blood-sugar control and promote good gut health. They also may help protect against diseases like heart disease.

1 Preheat the oven to 200°C (400°F).

2 Scatter the kale over a roasting tray, add a drizzle of the oil, season with salt and pepper and toss. Roast for 6-7 minutes, then toss with the sesame seeds and roast for a further 5-6 minutes until crisp. Drain on kitchen towel.

3 Meanwhile, heat half the remaining oil in a large pan over medium-low heat and gently fry the onion, seasoned with a little sea salt, for 10 minutes until really soft.

4 Add the rest of the oil to the pan. Increase the heat, add the mushroom and fry until the mushroom is golden brown and the onion is sticky. Add the chilli and vinegar, season well and cook for a minute more, then add the soy sauce.

5 Toast the bread and top with the mushroom and some of the crispy kale. Drizzle with extra virgin olive oil and serve.

Tips

The extra crispy kale will keep in an airtight container for 3-4 days. If you want to, you can also scatter with crumbled feta cheese.

Soups

Red cabbage soup

Serves 6
Ready in 40 minutes

VO GF

This is one of my signature dishes, and I love the vibrant purple colour. I got the inspiration for this soup when I tasted something similar at a delightful bistro called Re-bio in Rome. Cruciferous veggies like red cabbage help to regulate the healthy metabolism of oestrogens in the liver. Red cabbage is a double hero ingredient for me as it's also high in anthocyanins, antioxidants that are good for your skin.

2 tbsp olive oil
1 red onion, finely sliced
1 large leek, finely sliced
4 sprigs of fresh thyme, leaves stripped, or ½ tsp dried
500g (1lb 2oz) red cabbage, shredded
350g (12oz) floury potatoes, peeled and chopped
800ml (3¼ cups) fresh vegetable stock or Chicken bone broth (see page 227) (or use 2 gluten-free low-sodium stock cubes)
6 tsp natural yoghurt or crème fraîche

1 Heat the oil in a deep pan over a medium heat and gently fry the onion and leek with the thyme for 10 minutes until really softened.

2 Add the cabbage, potato and stock. Season and simmer gently for 20 minutes until the potato is tender.

3 Blend with a stick blender until smooth, then serve with a drizzle of yoghurt or crème fraîche and plenty of black pepper.

healthy skin | hormone balance

HELPS WITH

Tips ─────────────

This soup freezes brilliantly in batches – just defrost and reheat. Top with a small handful of pumpkin seeds (pepitas) and/or serve with a slice of seeded or sourdough bread (gluten free, if you prefer).

Anti-inflammatory carrot and ginger soup

Serves 6
Ready in 25 minutes

V GF

This is comfort in a bowl. It's wonderful for when you're feeling run-down as it's uber nourishing. The hero ingredients here are all the anti-inflammatory spices and herbs. I love the kick of ginger the most. Through eating prebiotics, found in ginger and plant foods in general, you can support the anti-inflammatory benefits of your gut microbiome.

1 tbsp olive oil or Garlic oil
   (see page 224)
1 red onion, finely chopped
2 celery sticks, chopped
2cm (¾ inch) piece of fresh
   turmeric, peeled and grated,
   or ¼ tsp ground
3cm (1¼ inch) piece of fresh
   ginger, peeled and grated
500g (1lb 2oz) carrots, peeled
   and chopped
1 x 400g (14oz) tin chickpeas,
   drained and rinsed
750ml (3 cups) fresh
   vegetable stock (or use
   2 gluten-free low-sodium
   stock cubes)
2 tbsp kefir yoghurt or crème
   fraiche
Small handful of fresh
   coriander (cilantro) leaves,
   (optional)
Small handful of pumpkin
   seeds (pepitas)

1 Heat the oil in a saucepan over a medium heat and gently fry the onion and celery for 5 minutes, until softened but not coloured.

2 Add the turmeric, ginger and carrot and fry briefly, then add the chickpeas and vegetable stock. Season with salt and pepper and bring to the boil, then reduce to a simmer and cook for 10–12 minutes until the carrot is tender.

3 Whizz with a stick blender or in a food processor until smooth, then serve with the yoghurt or crème fraiche, a few coriander leaves, if using, the pumpkin seeds and plenty of black pepper.

Tips

Freeze the soup in portions and defrost and reheat when needed. Serve with a slice of seeded or sourdough bread (gluten free, if preferred).

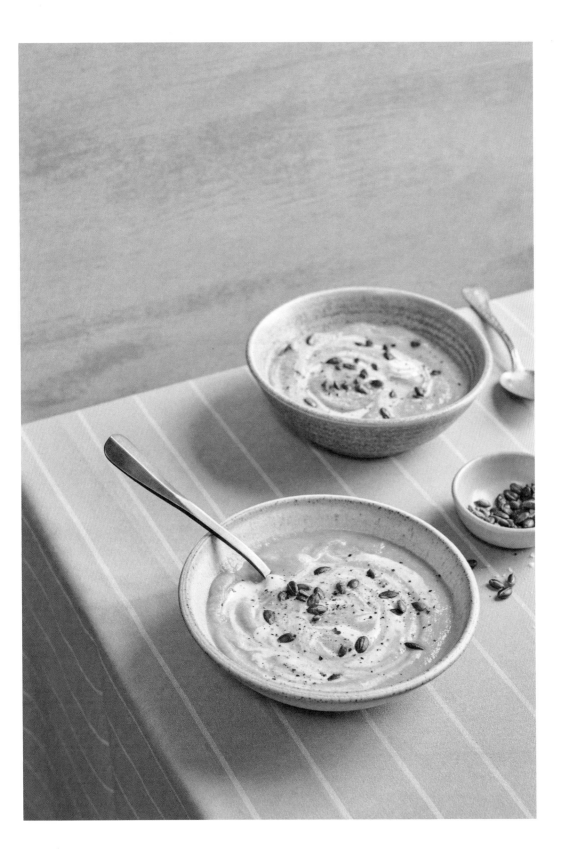

Roasted red pepper, tomato and bean soup

Serves 4–6
Ready in 45 minutes

VO GF

Soups make a fantastic lunch, but they tend to be low in protein. In this recipe, the beans are the hero ingredient, as they not only push up the protein and fibre content, they are also a good source of vitamin B6. Vitamin B6 supports liver function, can help balance our hormones and also helps with mood. Topping the soup with kefir helps support a balanced microbiome.

2 red peppers (capsicums), deseeded and quartered
200g (7oz) cherry tomatoes, halved
1 red onion, cut into wedges
2 tbsp olive oil
10 fresh sage leaves, plus a few extra, to serve
1 x 400g (14oz) tin white beans (such as butter or cannellini), drained and rinsed
450ml (generous 1¾ cups) fresh vegetable stock or Chicken bone broth (see page 227) (or use a gluten-free low-sodium stock cube)
4 tbsp kefir yoghurt

1 Preheat the oven to 200ºC (400ºF).

2 Toss the pepper, tomato and onion in a roasting tin with the olive oil and sage. Season with salt and pepper and roast for 25-30 minutes until tender and starting to become golden.

3 Add the beans and roast for 10 minutes more.

4 Set aside a third of the beans. Transfer the rest of the mixture to a saucepan and add the stock. Bring to a simmer, then blitz with a stick blender.

5 Serve in bowls scattered with the reserved roasted beans, sage leaves, a drizzle of kefir and some black pepper.

Tips

Fry a few extra sage leaves in olive oil for a minute until crisp, drain on kitchen towel and use as a garnish.
Serve with a slice of seeded, sourdough or gluten-free bread.

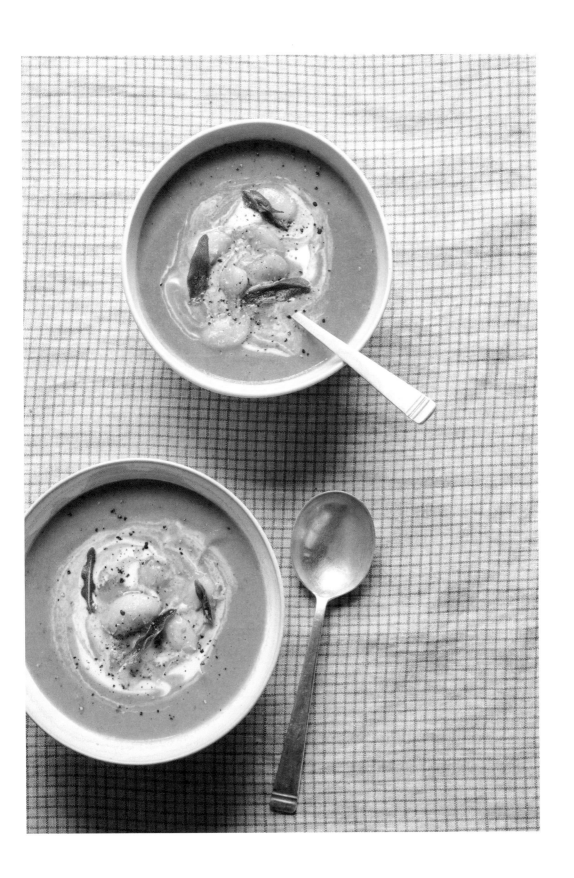

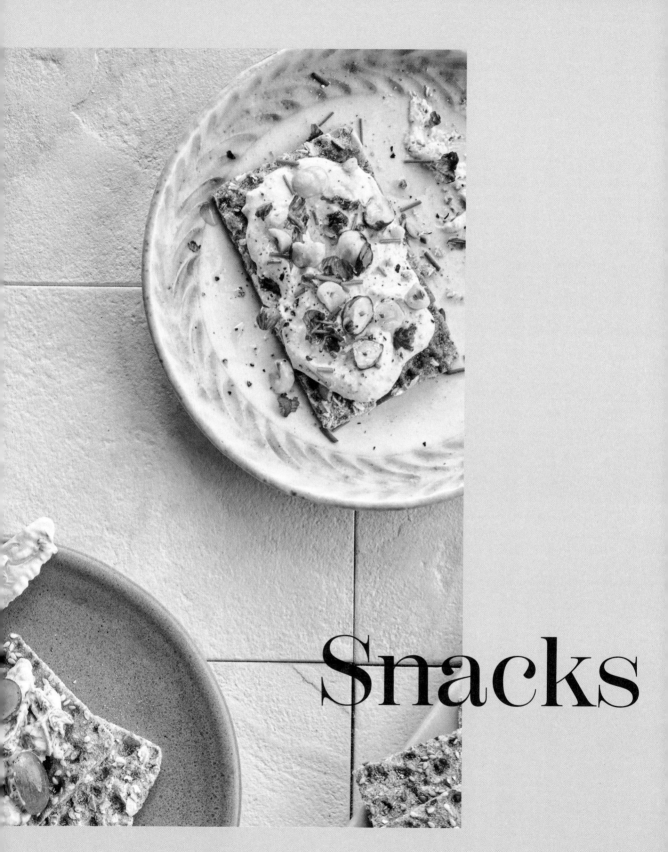

Snacks

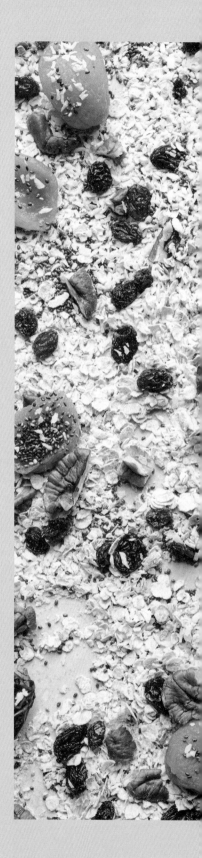

If you're a snacker, that's fine. The key is to be mindful with your snacking and snack smart. This means a little bit of preparation to make sure you have the good stuff on hand. A balanced snack should always contain some protein and some fibre. This snack section gives you a selection of healthy and balanced snacks, which can be eaten regularly.

Crispy roast chickpeas

Makes 600g (1lb 5oz)
Ready in 1 hour

VG GF

2 x 400g (14oz) tins chickpeas,
  drained and rinsed
1 tbsp olive oil
Good pinch of cayenne
  pepper
1 tsp ground cumin
½ tsp ground coriander
Good pinch of sumac

This is your healthy alternative to crisps. Legumes like chickpeas are nature's mixed meal. They contain both protein and carbs, making than naturally low glycaemic index and a great snack option. Adding spices gives flavour and adds an anti-inflammatory boost.

1 Preheat the oven to 200°C (400°F).

2 Dry the chickpeas really well by patting them with paper towel. Place them in a roasting tin and toss with the rest of the ingredients. Season with salt and pepper, then roast for 50 minutes, turning occasionally, until golden and crispy. Season with some sea salt and allow to cool.

Tips

You can also add harissa paste, zaatar, curry powder or chipotle. These will keep for 1–2 days in an airtight container.

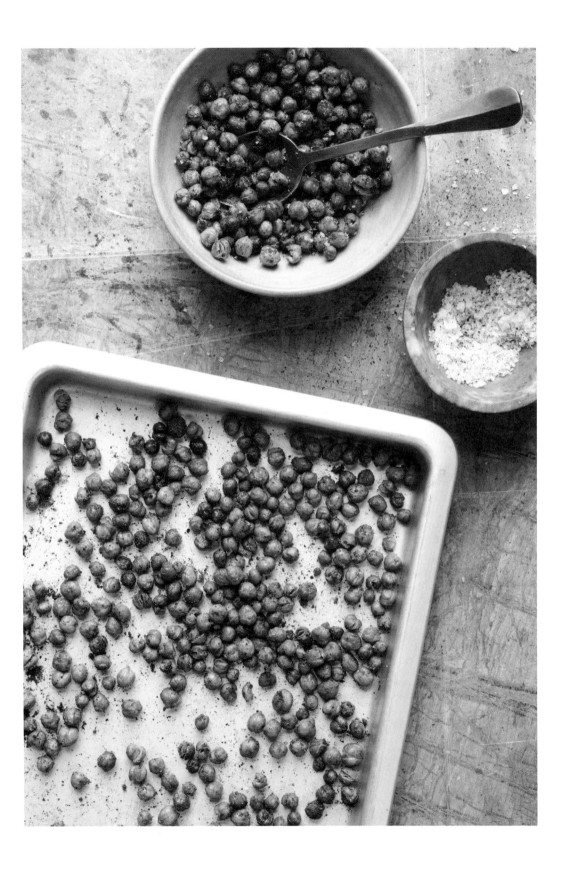

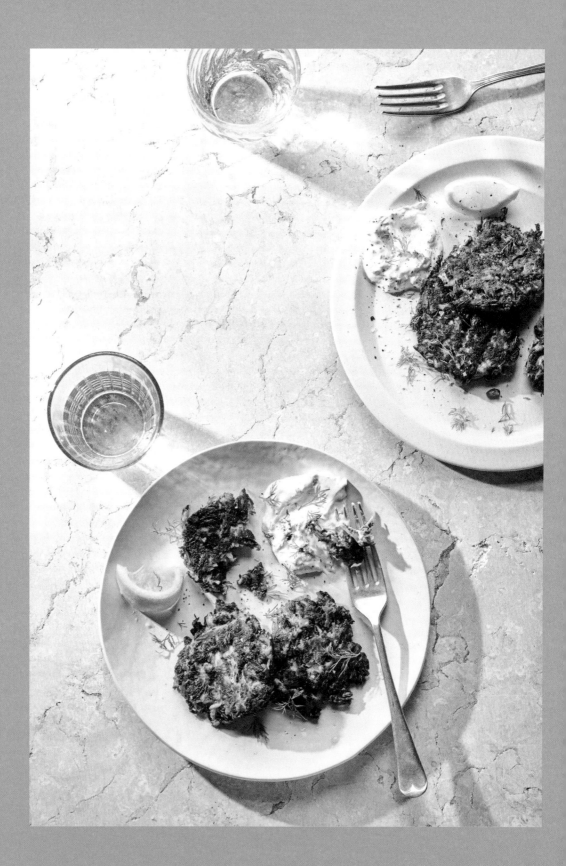

Tuna 'polpette'

Makes 12 small fritters
Ready in 30 minutes

GF

Polpette means 'meatball' in Italian. The recipe for traditional Italian meatballs uses breadcrumbs, which gives them their ball-like shape. To make these more of a menopause-friendly snack, I've omitted the breadcrumbs, so they are more like fritters. They're loaded with protein and are utterly delicious. The hero ingredient is cottage cheese. Approximately 70 per cent of the calories in cottage cheese are from protein. Protein-rich foods play an important role in keeping you fuller for longer – which is key when it comes to snacking.

2 tbsp olive oil
1 small onion, finely chopped
200g (7oz) baby spinach
1 tsp fennel seeds
1 x 200g (7oz) tin top-quality
  tuna in olive oil, drained
1 medium egg
100g (⅓ cup) cottage cheese
1 tbsp capers, chopped
1 heaped tbsp ground
  flaxseed
2 tbsp chopped fresh dill,
  or 1 tsp dried

Dipping sauce
100g (⅓ cup) Greek yoghurt
  or thick kefir yoghurt
Zest of 1 lemon
1 tbsp chopped fresh dill

1 Heat a little drizzle of the oil in a frying pan over a medium-low heat and gently fry the onion for 5 minutes until softened. Add the spinach and fennel seeds and allow the spinach to wilt. Transfer to a bowl and allow to cool a little.

2 Once cool enough to handle, drain off any excess liquid and squeeze dry, then roughly chop. Mix with the tuna, egg, cottage cheese, capers, flaxseed and dill. Season well with sea salt and freshly ground black pepper.

3 Heat the remaining oil in the pan over a medium heat and fry tablespoonfuls of the mixture, in batches, pressing down lightly, for 1–2 minutes. Flip and fry on the other side for another 1–2 minutes until golden all over.

4 To make the dipping sauce, mix the yoghurt in a bowl with the lemon zest, dill and some salt and pepper. Serve with the fritters.

Tips

These will keep in the fridge for 4–5 days in a sealed container, so you can just grab them as you need them. Heat them briefly in a hot oven or dry frying pan to warm up before serving.

Crispbread toppings

When you get home from work, dinner is not yet made and you are tired and peckish, it's tempting to reach for the kids' leftovers or whatever you can get your hands on in the cupboards or the fridge. Be prepared! These snack options are there to help you fill that gap and nourish you. You can serve them on a wholegrain cracker bread or with veggie crudités.

Walnut and spinach yoghurt spread

Makes 200g (7oz) spread
(4–6 servings)
Ready in 20 minutes

V   GF

80g (⅔ cup) walnuts
120g (4¼oz) baby spinach
½ tsp ground coriander
Good pinch of chilli flakes
150g (generous ½ cup) thick
   Greek yoghurt
1 tsp finely chopped fresh
   mint, or a pinch of dried
Squeeze of lemon juice
   (optional)
Red grapes, sliced, to serve
Extra virgin olive oil, to drizzle

Walnuts are sometimes referred to as the 'king of the nuts' as they possess fantastic nutritional qualities. They are high in anti-inflammatory omega-3s and they are also a great source of magnesium. Magnesium plays a role in the production of the neurotransmitter that regulates mood. While this recipe may sound like a weird combo, I promise you it's good. You can use it as a spread or a dip.

1 Toast the walnuts in a dry frying pan over a low heat for 5 minutes until golden. When cooled, chop them quite finely, but leave some larger pieces, and place in a mixing bowl.

2 Add the spinach to the pan along with a splash of water. Allow to wilt, then remove from heat and squeeze out as much liquid as you can. Roughly chop and add to the walnuts along with the spices, yoghurt and mint. Mix well. Season with sea salt and freshly ground black pepper, adding a squeeze of lemon, if using.

3 Serve on crispbreads, topped with sliced grapes and a drizzle of extra virgin olive oil.

Tip

This would also be great served as a side with grilled chicken.

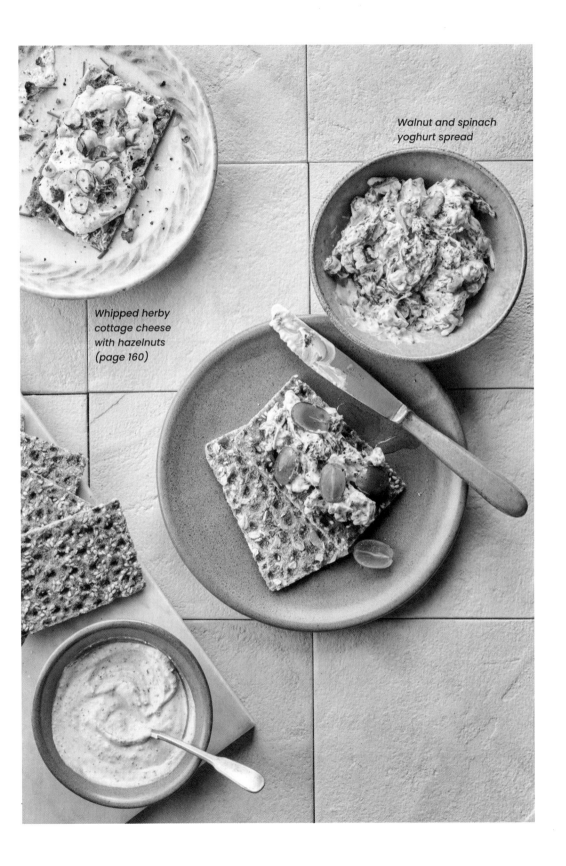

Walnut and spinach
yoghurt spread

Whipped herby
cottage cheese
with hazelnuts
(page 160)

Whipped herby cottage cheese with hazelnuts

mood regulation

HELPS WITH

Makes 200g (7oz) spread
(4–6 servings)
Ready in 10 minutes

V GF

I love a good dip, especially one that's as nutrient dense as this one. It contains protein from the cottage cheese, healthy fats and fibre from the hazelnuts and lots of phytonutrients. The herbs help take it to another level, in terms of taste and nutrients.

200g (¾ cup) cottage cheese
  (full-fat)
1 tbsp finely chopped fresh
  chives
1 tbsp finely chopped fresh dill
1 tbsp finely chopped fresh
  flat-leaf parsley
Topping
40g (⅓ cup) chopped toasted
  hazelnuts
1 tbsp finely chopped fresh
  chives
Extra virgin olive oil, to drizzle

1 In a small food processor, whizz the cottage cheese with the herbs and some sea salt and freshly ground black pepper.

2 Serve on crispbreads with the hazelnuts and chives scattered over the top and finish with a drizzle of extra virgin olive oil.

Tip

Try using almonds instead of hazelnuts.

Hummus 3 ways

Once you start making your own hummus, you won't go back to using shop-bought. Nutty, creamy and delicious, homemade hummus is easy and rustic and you can play around with flavours. I love the vibrant colours – phytonutrient power! With legumes and beans at the heart of each of my recipes, they are fantastic sources of plant-based protein and fibre. Eat as a dip, spread on sandwiches or add to salads for a flavour boost.

Classic hummus

Makes 250g (9oz) hummus
Ready in 15 minutes

VG GF

You have to have a classic hummus recipe up your sleeve. Being naturally high in fibre and protein, chickpeas help with blood-sugar control and digestive health, both of which are important things to keep on top of during the menopause.

1 x 400g (14oz) tin chickpeas, drained and rinsed
1 heaped tbsp tahini
Generous pinch of ground cumin
1 clove garlic (optional)
Finely grated zest of a lemon and a good squeeze of juice
4 tbsp extra virgin olive oil, plus extra, to drizzle
Good pinch of sumac

1 Put the chickpeas into a food processor (setting aside a handful for garnish). Add the tahini, cumin, garlic, if using, lemon zest and juice and olive oil. Blitz together. Season to taste with sea salt and freshly ground black pepper, adding more lemon juice if needed. You can loosen with a little water if you like a thinner consistency.

2 Scatter with the reserved chickpeas, drizzle with extra virgin olive oil and scatter with the sumac before serving.

Tip

If you have time, try using dried chickpeas. Soak 125g (⅔ cup) dried chickpeas overnight or for up to 24 hours. Drain, cover with water and a good pinch of salt and simmer gently until very tender (the cooking time varies, so start checking after about 40 minutes). Drain and cool, then add to the food processor with the other ingredients.

Edamame hummus

Makes 200g (7oz) hummus
Ready in 15 minutes

VG GF

150g (5½oz) frozen
  edamame beans
50g (2oz) baby spinach
Large handful of fresh
  basil leaves
1 tbsp tahini
2-3 tbsp Garlic oil (see
  page 224)
Good squeeze of lemon juice
Black and white sesame
  seeds, to sprinkle

Some studies suggest that soy isoflavones (found in edamame beans) may help reduce the hot flushes and night sweats that many women have during menopause. They are also a fantastic source of plant-based protein and won't bloat you as much as some other beans.

1 In a pan of boiling water, blanch the edamame and spinach until the spinach is wilted and the edamame are tender. Drain and run under cold water to cool, then squeeze out as much moisture as possible from the spinach.

2 Put into a small food processor and blitz with the basil, tahini, garlic oil and lemon juice. Season to taste and serve scattered with sesame seeds.

Tip

Keeps in the fridge for up to a week.

Beetroot hummus

Makes 300g (10½oz) hummus
Ready in 50 minutes

GF

1 medium beetroot (about
   150g/5½oz)
1 x 400g (14oz) tin white beans,
   drained and rinsed
1 tbsp tahini
Juice of ½ a lemon
2 tbsp extra virgin olive oil,
   plus extra, to drizzle

Topping
2 tbsp pumpkin seeds
   (pepitas), toasted
75g (2½oz) feta cheese,
   crumbled

Beetroot contains dietary nitrates that may help to dilate blood vessels. They are a good addition to your diet, particularly if you suffer from hot flushes. Beetroot also contains antioxidants called betalains, which have anti-inflammatory properties.

1 Preheat the oven to 200°C (400°F).

2 Wrap the beetroot in foil and roast for 40 minutes until really tender. Allow to cool a little, then peel and discard the skin and roughly chop the flesh.

3 In a food processor, whizz together the beetroot and beans, then add the tahini, lemon juice and oil and blend. Season to taste with sea salt and freshly ground black pepper.

4 Toast the pumpkin seeds in a dry pan until they burst.

5 Serve the hummus scattered with feta cheese, toasted pumpkin seeds and a drizzle of extra virgin olive oil.

Tips

If you want to speed things up, use ready-roasted beetroot. The colour won't be quite so electric, but it will taste just as delicious. You can also roast your beetroot in advance and keep it in the fridge for up to a week.

No-bake energy balls 3 ways

These are the ultimate easy no-bake energy balls. There's no added sugar, yet they all have a natural sweetness that hits the spot. Make a batch and snack smart for the whole week! Note: One serve is two balls.

Carrot cake balls with apricot and ginger

Makes 10-12 balls
Ready in 20 minutes, plus chilling

VG GF

Where possible, I will always sneak some vegetables into my energy balls, and there is a little fibre hit from the carrot here. However, my favourite thing about these balls is the addition of the ginger. There is not enough research on ginger and menopause. However, based on what research there is, ginger is linked to reduced inflammation, better digestion and positive effects on general wellbeing.

125g (¾ cup) dates
100ml (scant ½ cup) boiling water
1 large (about 130g/4½oz) carrot, coarsely grated
50g (scant ½ cup) walnuts
3 tbsp ground flaxseed
60g (⅓ cup) dried apricots
1 tsp ground ginger
½ tsp ground cinnamon

1 Soak the dates in the boiling water for 10 minutes, then scoop out (reserving the water). Place in a food processor along with the rest of the ingredients and blitz. Add enough of the soaking water to bring it all together.

2 Shape the mixture into 10–12 walnut-sized balls and chill on a lined baking sheet for at least 1 hour.

Tip

These will keep in the fridge for a week, or you can freeze them and defrost a few at a time.

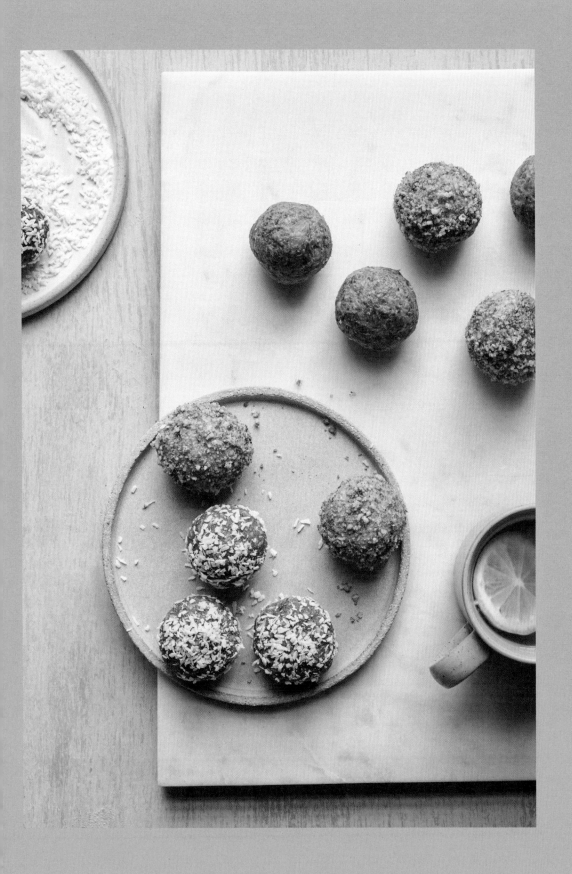

Peanut butter and chocolate-chip balls

mood regulation | sugar cravings

HELPS WITH

Makes 10-12 balls
Ready in 15 minutes, plus chilling

VG GF

150g (5½oz) cooked quinoa
4 tbsp peanut butter
2 tbsp chia seeds
2 tbsp maple syrup
30g (⅓ cup) desiccated
   coconut, plus extra for rolling
50g (⅓ cup) dark (at least
   70%) chocolate chips

I had the idea for these when I was making some energy balls and I realised I had some leftover quinoa lurking in the fridge. Quinoa ticks the boxes for protein and fibre. When I am craving something that is a little indulgent but won't derail my blood-sugar levels, these hit the spot. Dark chocolate is a fantastic source of magnesium. This mineral helps raise your mood-regulating hormone serotonin, which is why eating these balls perks you up!

1 Put the ingredients into a small food processor and blitz together. Shape into 10–12 balls and roll in extra desiccated coconut. Chill on a lined baking sheet for at least 1 hour.

Tips

You can also coat these in a layer of cocoa powder.
They keep in an airtight container for 2–3 days.

Pumpkin, cinnamon and raisin balls

Makes 10 balls
Ready in 25 minutes,
plus chilling

VG GF

150g (5½oz) pumpkin (or
squash), peeled, deseeded
and cut into chunks
60g (generous ½ cup)
gluten-free rolled oats
40g (scant ½ cup) pecans
3 tbsp almond butter
50g (¼ cup) raisins
1 tsp ground cinnamon

Not only does adding pumpkin bring more fibre to these balls, it also adds some vitamin A, which supports healthy, glowing skin. Be generous with the cinnamon here as this sweet-smelling spice has been linked to helping regulate blood-sugar control. It's not a magic bullet, but it's definitely a good addition during the menopause.

1 Steam the pumpkin in a steamer for 10 minutes until really tender. Mash and set aside to cool.

2 Put the oats and nuts into a small food processor and blitz until coarsely ground. Add the pumpkin purée and the rest of the ingredients and blitz until it comes together.

3 Shape into 10 balls and chill on a lined baking sheet for at least 1 hour.

Tips

You can use tinned unsweetened pumpkin purée to speed this up. They keep in an airtight container for 2–3 days.

Chia puddings 2 ways

I make these chia pots regularly as an afternoon snack. I use them as a little, yet massively delicious, fibre and probiotic boost. Chia seeds are a fantastic source of fibre and kefir contains live bacteria. Raspberries and blueberries are bursting with antioxidants, which reduce inflammation. It's always best to have a variety of berries, so feel free to swap them for your favourite berries or other fruits! You can also try other yoghurts.

Coconut and raspberry

Makes 2 puddings
Ready in 10 minutes, plus chilling

V GF

100ml (scant ½ cup) kefir
120g (½ cup) coconut yoghurt
100g (scant 1 cup) raspberries,
  plus a few to scatter
1 tbsp honey
2 tbsp chia seeds
1 tbsp desiccated coconut

1 In a blender, whizz together the kefir, yoghurt, raspberries and honey. Mix in the chia seeds and spoon into two glasses.

2 Top with the remaining raspberries and coconut and chill for at least 2 hours but ideally overnight.

Lemon and blueberry

Makes 2 puddings
Ready in 15 minutes, plus chilling

V GF

100g (⅔ cup) blueberries,
  plus a few to scatter
Finely grated zest of 1 lemon
  and a squeeze of juice
1 tbsp maple syrup
2 tbsp chia seeds
200ml (generous ¾ cup) kefir

1 Put the blueberries, lemon zest and juice and the syrup into a pan and cook over a medium heat for 3–4 minutes until the blueberries soften and become juicy. Allow to cool.

2 Mix the blueberries with the chia seeds and kefir, then spoon into two pots and chill for at least an hour. Top with the remaining blueberries to serve.

Tip

Replace the lemon with an orange and add a pinch of ground cinnamon for a twist.

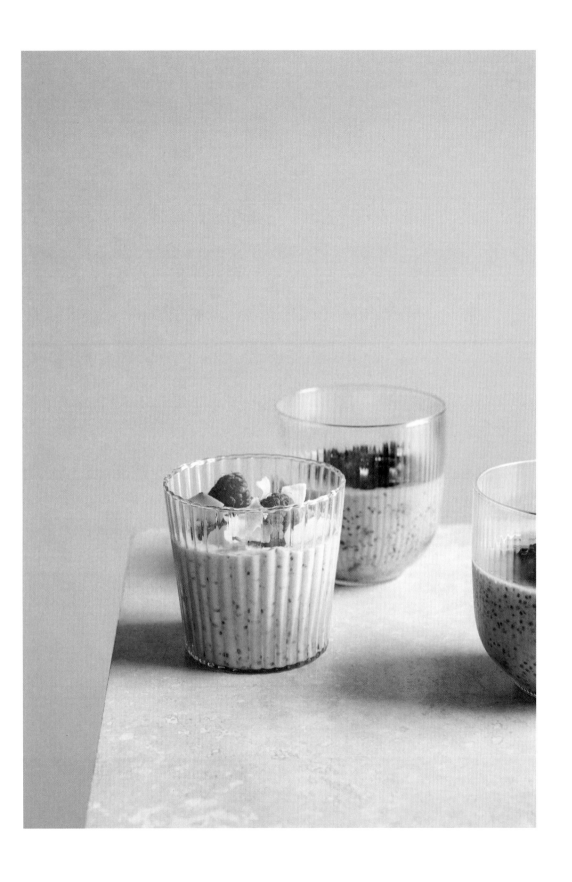

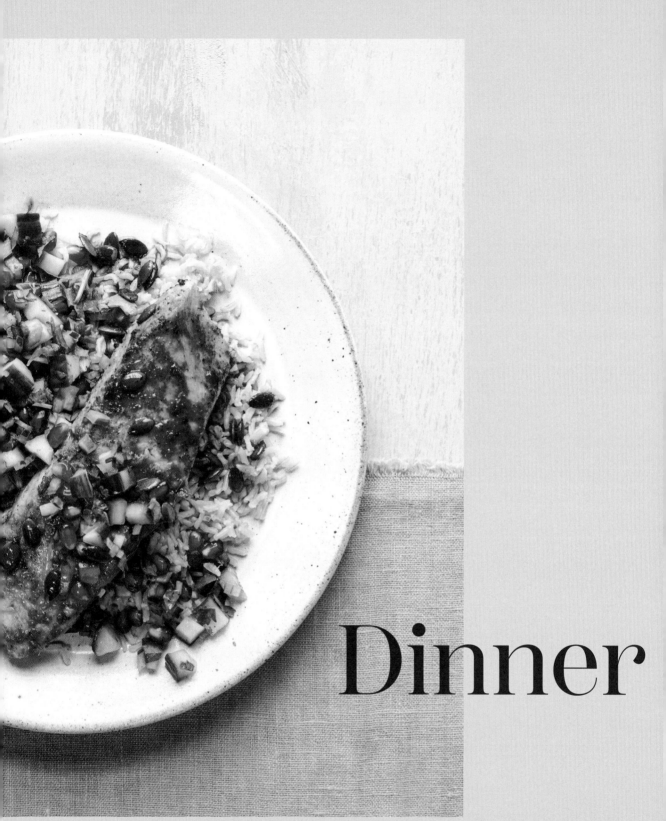

Dinner

These midweek dinners are easy and quick to make, as most of us are time-poor during the week, and they are designed to be family-friendly, so you don't have to cook different meals for different family members. Remember, though, the timing of your starchy carbohydrates is important during the menopause, particularly if you're looking to manage your weight. If you are, you may be better off keeping dinner low in starchy carbohydrates and focusing on the veggies (fibrous carbs) and some lean protein. Where the recipe contains some starchy carbohydrates, simply serve to your family members but don't put any on your own plate. You can still have the rest of the meal. I have not stipulated the salt intake, so you can season as you desire, but eating less salt helps ease water retention. Be generous with the pepper. Go easy on the salt.

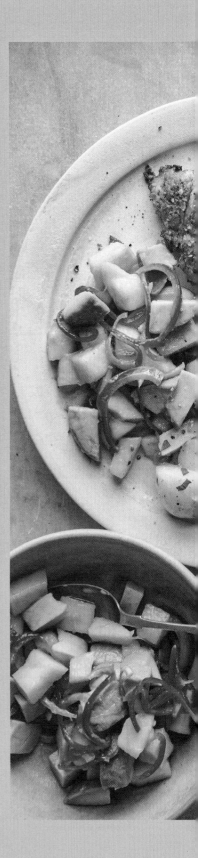

Gut-healing chicken korma

Serves 4–6
Ready in 40 minutes

GF

2 tbsp olive oil
1 red onion, coarsely grated
2 cloves garlic, whole
  (optional)
2–3cm (¾–1¼ inch) piece
  of fresh ginger, peeled
  and grated
1 tsp ground turmeric
2 tsp ground cumin
1 tsp ground coriander
½ tsp fenugreek seeds
¼ tsp chilli powder
1 tbsp tomato paste
  (concentrated purée)
4 chicken breasts, sliced into
  bite-sized pieces
2 tbsp ground almonds
400ml (1½ cups) Chicken bone
  broth (see page 227) or fresh
  chicken stock (or use a
  gluten-free low-sodium
  stock cube)
200g (7oz) spring greens,
  finely shredded
100g (⅓ cup) natural yoghurt
Large handful of fresh
  coriander (cilantro),
  chopped (optional)

I love this recipe. It takes me home and wraps me up in a warm blanket. Most kormas tend to be super rich, with lots of cream added – which doesn't help your gut bacteria thrive. I've replaced the cream with ground almonds and yoghurt, so this is better for your gut bugs, yet still deliciously creamy. The herbs and spices are the hero ingredients in this recipe as each one contains different phytonutrients that nourish your microbiome. You get over 10 plant points here – your gut is celebrating!

1 Heat the olive oil in a frying pan over a medium-high heat. Add the onion and fry for 5 minutes, then add the garlic, if using, and ginger and fry for 5 minutes more until soft and fragrant.

2 Add the spices, fenugreek seeds, chilli powder and tomato paste and cook for 2–3 minutes, then add the chicken.

3 Stir in the ground almonds and broth and season well with sea salt and freshly ground black pepper. Reduce heat and simmer gently for 20 minutes until the chicken is cooked through and the sauce has reduced.

4 Add the greens and yoghurt and cook gently until the greens are just wilted. Remove the garlic, if using, and serve scattered with fresh coriander, if you like.

Tips

If you want to speed things up, you could use 2 tbsp korma curry paste instead of the spices. The curry can also be frozen in portions for up to 3 months, so double up this recipe and freeze half (defrost fully before reheating).
Serve with brown or red rice, or on a bed of steamed veggies if you're cutting out starchy carbs at dinner.

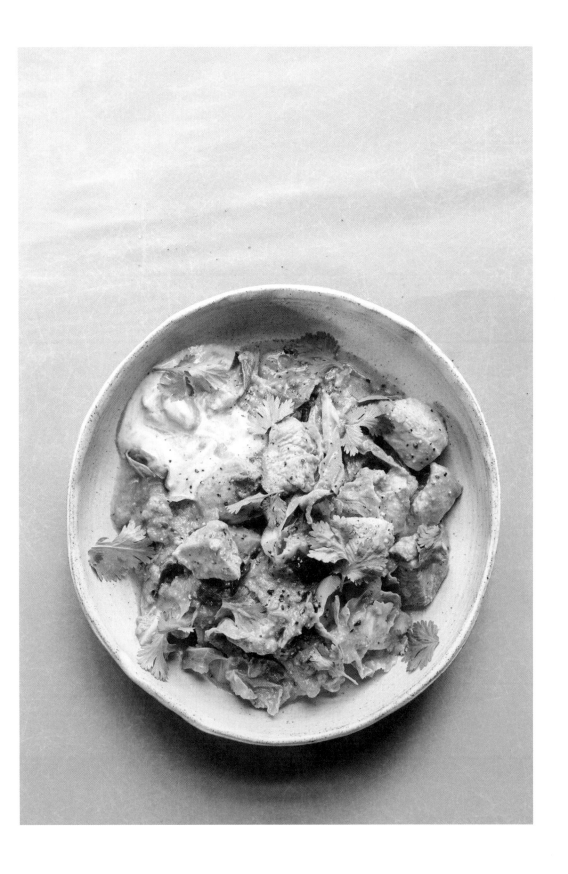

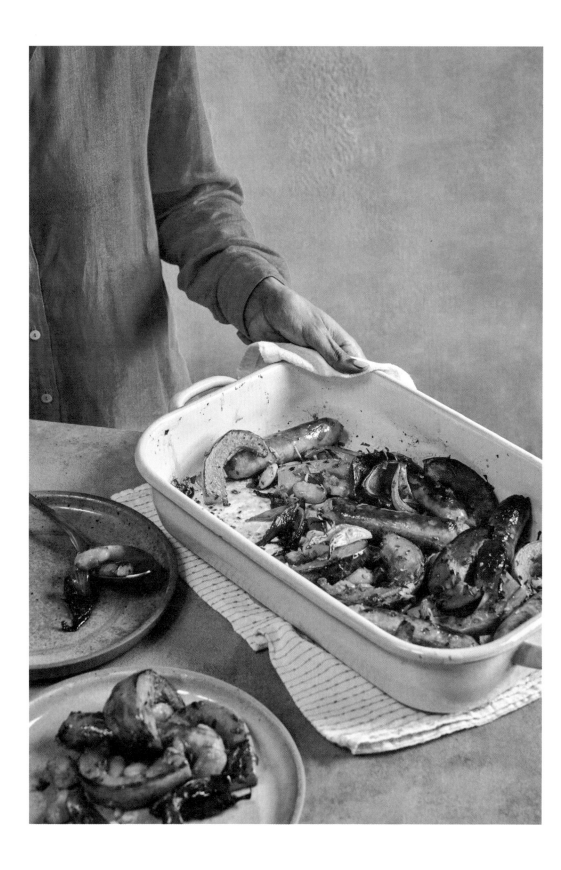

One-pan harissa sausage and bean bake

Serves 4
Ready in 50 minutes

DF GFO

One-pan meals have become a staple during my week. They are quick and easy, you can mix them up to ensure you get the nutrition you need ... and with just one pan to clean? I'm in! This recipe is balanced as it contains fibre (veggies), protein (your sausages of choice) and starchy and fibrous carbs (beans). If you want to make it lower in starchy carbohydrates, you can omit the beans and add more veggies. Pumpkin is the hero ingredient here. Pumpkins are high in fibre and lower in carbs than you may think. They contain only half the carbs found in sweet potatoes or normal potatoes, for example.

2 tbsp olive oil
8 sausages of your choice (gluten free if preferred)
1 red onion, cut into wedges
700g (1lb 9oz) pumpkin or butternut squash, cut into medium chunks
1 tbsp harissa paste
1 tsp cumin seeds
1 x 400g (14oz) tin white beans, drained and rinsed
75 ml (⅓ cup) fresh vegetable stock (or use a gluten-free low-sodium stock cube)
Handful of fresh flat-leaf parsley, finely chopped

1 Preheat the oven to 200°C (400°F).

2 Heat the olive oil in a large frying pan over a medium-high heat and briefly fry the sausages just enough to get the browning started, but not to cook them.

3 Transfer the sausages to a large roasting dish. Add the red onion, pumpkin, harissa paste and cumin seeds and toss together with sea salt and freshly ground black pepper.

4 Roast for 30 minutes, then stir in the beans and stock and roast for 10 minutes more. Scatter with parsley and serve.

Tip

You can serve this topped with crumbled feta cheese and toasted pumpkin seeds (pepitas).

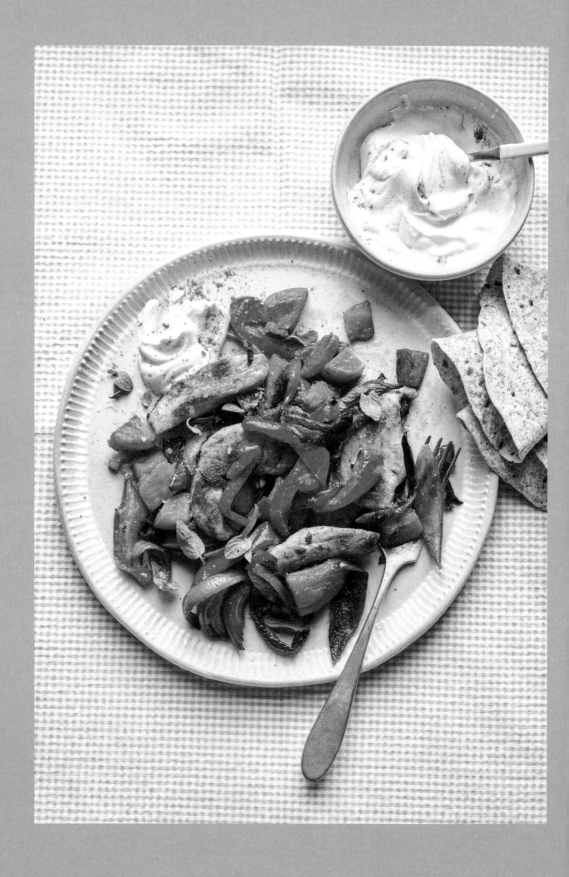

Chicken fajita tray bake

Serves 4
Ready in 1 hour

GFO

This is one of my favourite recipes in the book. I love the spice mix as it's delicious and doesn't have the salt and sugar you find in shop-bought varieties. The star ingredient in this recipe for me is the red onion. You will notice I use red onions in a lot of my recipes. This is because they are often overlooked but are a nutritional powerhouse! They are one of the highest natural sources of quercetin, which lowers inflammation. Cooling inflammation is essential for a healthy menopause transition.

2 large chicken breasts (about 350g/12oz), cut into chunks
2 large sweet potatoes, peeled and cut into cubes
1 large red onion, cut into wedges
2 red peppers (capsicums), deseeded and cut into medium strips
2 tbsp olive oil
1 tsp ground cumin
5 sprigs of fresh oregano, leaves stripped, or 1 tsp dried
1 tsp hot smoked paprika
Good pinch of cayenne pepper
Simple flatbreads (see page 224), to serve (optional)
Natural yoghurt, to serve

1 Preheat the oven to 200°C (400°F).

2 Toss together the chicken, sweet potato, red onion and pepper in a large roasting tin.

3 Drizzle with the olive oil and toss with all the spices and herbs. Season well with sea salt and freshly ground black pepper.

4 Roast for 40–45 minutes, stirring once or twice.

5 Serve the fajita mix with flatbreads, if using, and a dollop of yoghurt.

Tips

If you want to simplify this, you can use a fajita seasoning instead of the spices.
You can also serve this with wraps, rice or, for a low-carb option, try seaweed sheets or romaine lettuce leaves!

Halloumi and veg tray bake

Serves 4
Ready in 55 minutes

V   GF

Halloumi makes this easy veggie tray bake feel like a real treat. This recipe is a fantastic way to get in all your veggies, it's full of colour and variety, and your gut bugs will appreciate the diversity. I've used Mediterranean veggies, however you can add whatever veggies are in your fridge; it's a great way to reduce waste. Throw in a handful of edamame beans to further boost the protein content.

1 aubergine (eggplant), cut into 2cm (¾ inch) chunks
1 courgette (zucchini), thickly sliced
1 red pepper (capsicum), deseeded and sliced
1 red onion, cut into wedges
1 tbsp harissa paste
2 tbsp olive oil
250g (9oz) halloumi, sliced
2 tsp honey
100g (¾ cup) black olives
50g (2oz) wild rocket (arugula)

1 Preheat the oven to 200ºC (400ºF).

2 Toss together the aubergine, courgette, red pepper and onion in a large roasting tin with the harissa paste and olive oil.

3 Season well with sea salt and freshly ground black pepper. Roast for 35–40 minutes, turning once, until the vegetables are tender and lightly golden.

4 Nestle the slices of halloumi into the tray. Switch the oven to a medium-high grill setting and pop the tray back into the oven (or place under a medium-high grill) and grill for 5–6 minutes until the halloumi is golden brown.

5 Drizzle with the honey and scatter with the olives and rocket to serve.

Tips

Serve with Simple flatbreads (see page 224) or a side salad if you are going lower in carbs. Instead of the halloumi, you can scatter crumbled feta over before serving.

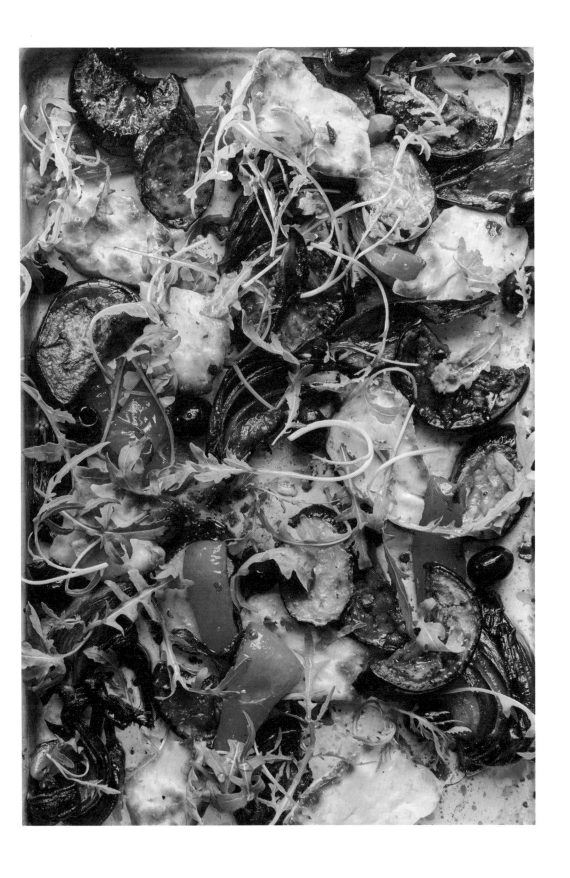

Speedy spinach and paneer coconut masala

Serves 4
Ready in 35 minutes

V GF

I love the flavour of garlic. However, having an irritable bowel means that it leaves me massively bloated. The menopause is linked with digestive changes, and many women experience bloating, so for all the recipes that need extra flavour, I have used garlic oil. This is a fantastic way to get the flavour into this delicious recipe minus the bloat. This is another one of my mama's recipes, but she used to make it with a tin of coconut cream! I have reduced that right down to 2 tablespoons, which means it still tastes as good as the original version but is much healthier for you.

2 tbsp Garlic oil (see page 224)
1 large red onion, finely chopped
2cm (¾ inch) piece of fresh ginger, peeled and grated
1 tbsp shop-bought tikka masala spice blend
200g (7oz) fresh tomatoes, chopped (or tinned)
90g (½ cup) red split lentils
250g (9oz) paneer, cubed
400ml (1½ cups) fresh vegetable stock (or use a gluten-free low-sodium stock cube)
120g (4¼oz) baby spinach
2 tbsp coconut cream

1 Heat the garlic oil in a frying pan over a medium heat and gently fry the onion for 5 minutes until it is softened and lightly golden.

2 Add the ginger, tikka masala spices and tomato and fry for 5 minutes, then add the lentils, paneer and vegetable stock. Season well with sea salt and freshly ground black pepper, then reduce the heat to low and simmer gently for 15 minutes.

3 Add the spinach and coconut cream and simmer for another 3–4 minutes until the spinach has wilted. Serve.

Tips

This freezes for up to 3 months, so double up this recipe for easy batch-cooking (defrost fully before reheating). Serve with red rice or, if you want a lower-carb option, on a bed of steamed veg.

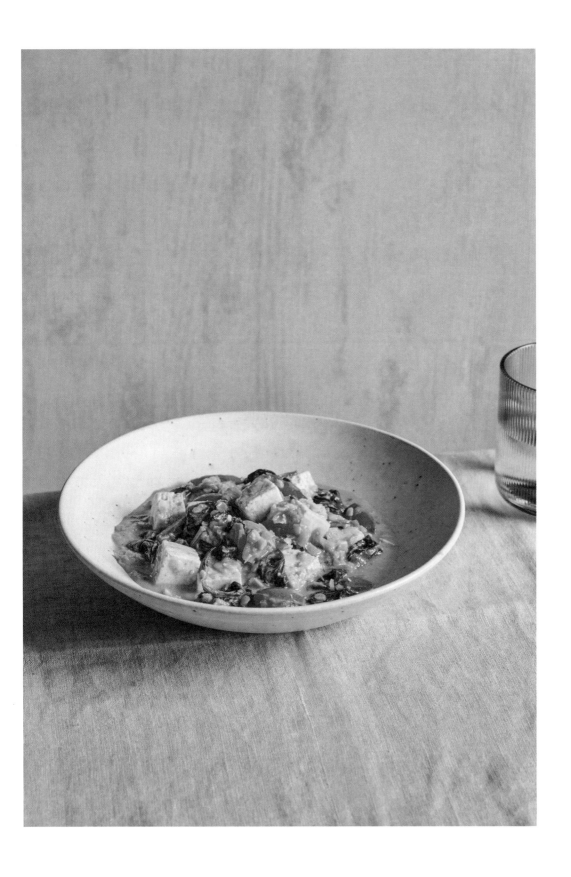

Chicken thigh cacciatore

Serves 4
Ready in 45 minutes

GF DF

2 tbsp olive oil
4 large or 8 small skin-on
  chicken thighs
1 red onion, finely sliced
2 celery sticks, finely sliced
200ml (generous ¾ cup) red
  wine (optional)
1 bay leaf
1 sprig of fresh rosemary,
  needles stripped, or ½ tsp
  dried
4 sprigs of fresh thyme, leaves
  stripped or ½ tsp dried
2 x 400g (14oz) tins cherry
  tomatoes
300ml (1¼ cups) Chicken bone
  broth (see page 227) or fresh
  chicken stock (or use a
  gluten-free low-sodium
  stock cube)
1 Savoy cabbage, leaves
  separated (discard any
  woody outer leaves)
120g (¾ cup) green olives
2 tbsp capers, drained and
  patted dry
Large handful of fresh flat-leaf
  parsley, finely chopped

Hearty and satisfying, this is a rustic Italian classic. Serve with veggies and sourdough bread or your favourite whole grain. I have added some cabbage because cruciferous veggies are an important addition for us ladies. They support our livers to work more efficiently, promoting hormone balance. Cabbage also contains antioxidants like sulforaphane and kaempferol, which may help reduce inflammation.

1 Heat half the olive oil in a large non-stick frying pan over a medium-high heat. Season the chicken with sea salt and freshly ground black pepper and fry for 8–10 minutes until browned all over. Transfer to a plate and set aside.

2 Heat the remaining oil in the frying pan over a medium heat. Add the onion and celery and gently fry for 5 minutes until softened.

3 Return the chicken to the pan, add the red wine and bubble for 3 minutes until reduced by half.

4 Add the herbs and cherry tomatoes, crushing the tomatoes lightly with the back of your spoon.

5 Season, then add the broth and simmer gently for 15 minutes. Add the whole cabbage leaves to the pan, cover and simmer gently for 5 minutes more until the leaves are softened and bright green.

6 Stir in the green olives and capers. Serve scattered with flat-leaf parsley.

Tip

Double up this recipe for an easy batch cook and freeze the finished dish for up to 3 months (defrost fully before reheating).

Red lentil crepe with mushrooms, egg and spinach

Serves 4
Ready in 30 minutes, plus overnight soaking

V GF

For a light dinner, I like to have something with egg. This is a lovely recipe, which you can enjoy all year round, that the whole family will love. Crepes are often made with flour, but I have swapped out the flour for red lentils to give you more protein and fibre – two important nutrients during the menopause. I also added some mushrooms as they are a wonderful menopause nutrition staple. Rich in fibre, they contain more protein than most veggies and are a powerful source of bio-active ingredients that support a good immune system.

120g (generous ½ cup) red split lentils
3 tbsp olive oil or Garlic oil (see page 224)
4 portobello mushrooms, sliced
Pinch of chilli flakes
150g (5½oz) baby spinach
150ml (generous ½ cup) water
1 tbsp chickpea flour (besan)
½ tsp ground turmeric
1 tsp ground cumin
1 tsp ground coriander
½ tsp baking powder
½ tsp fine sea salt
2 tbsp cottage cheese (or yoghurt)
4 medium eggs

1 Soak the lentils overnight in cold water.

2 Heat 1 tablespoon of the olive oil in a large pan over a high heat. Add the mushroom and chilli flakes and fry for 5 minutes until golden. Add the spinach and allow it to wilt, then season well. Set aside and keep warm.

3 Drain the lentils well, then put them into a food processor or blender and whizz with the water, chickpea flour, spices, baking powder, salt and cottage cheese.

4 Heat ½ teaspoon of the remaining oil in a 20cm (8-inch) non-stick frying pan over a medium-high heat. Once hot, add a ladleful of the lentil batter. Swirl the pan so the batter covers the base. Cook for 2–3 minutes until the edges are coming away and it is starting to crisp, then flip and cook for 2–3 minutes. Tip onto a warm plate and repeat with the rest of the mixture to make three more crepes, adding ½ teaspoon of oil for each.

5 Heat the remaining oil in a clean frying pan over a medium heat and fry the eggs until crispy.

6 Serve the crepes with the mushroom mixture and crispy eggs.

Tip

The crepes would also be delicious served with pan-fried paneer or the Speedy spinach and paneer coconut masala on page 180.

Healthy chicken cotoletta with mango and avo salsa

Serves 4
Ready in 35 minutes

Flaxseed is the one ingredient I probably eat every day and that I think every forty-plus woman should be adding to their diet. It is rich in omega-3 rand contains 100 times more lignans (a plant-based phytonutrient) than any other food out there. It's a great addition for healthy hormones. I was so impressed that I managed to sneak flaxseed into a classic Milanese speciality like this! Cotoletta is the Italian version of a schnitzel.

*4 small or 2 large
  chicken breasts
1 tbsp ground flaxseed
1 medium egg, whisked
60g (generous ½ cup) dried
  breadcrumbs
1 tbsp sesame seeds
20g (¼ cup) grated parmesan
1 tbsp olive oil*
Salsa
*1 large ripe mango
1 red onion, finely sliced
1 ripe avocado, diced
Juice of 1 lime*

1 Preheat the oven to 220°C (425°F).

2 With a rolling pin, flatten the chicken breasts between two pieces of parchment paper until about 5mm (¼ inch) thick.

3 Season the chicken with sea salt and freshly ground black pepper. Place the ground flaxseed in one bowl and the egg in another. Dip the chicken into the ground flaxseed, followed by the egg. In a third bowl, mix the breadcrumbs with the sesame seeds and cheese and coat the chicken in the mixture.

4 Place the coated chicken on a baking tray and drizzle with the olive oil. Bake for 15 minutes, then turn and bake for 5 minutes more until golden and crisp.

5 For the salsa, slice the flesh from the mango and finely dice, then toss with the red onion, avocado, lime juice and some seasoning.

6 Serve the chicken and salsa with sides of your choice.

Tips

You can use slices of pork tenderloin instead of the chicken or turkey. Serve with new potatoes or the Red cabbage slaw on page 216.

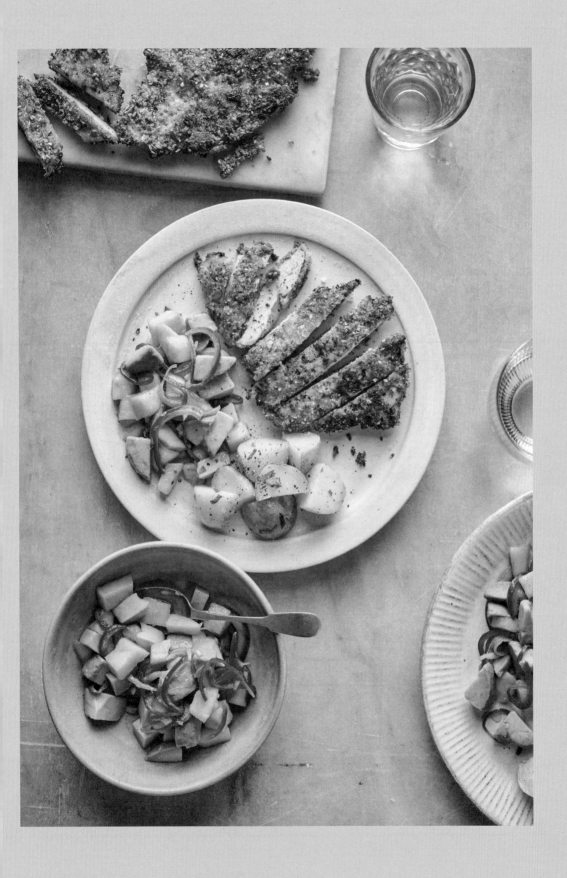

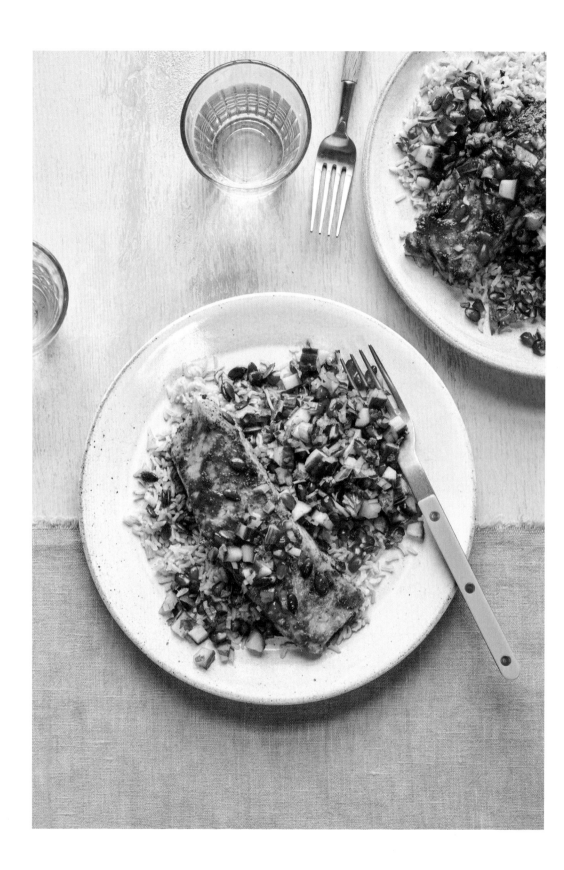

Crispy-crusted Thai-style salmon with salsa

Serves 4
Ready in 20 minutes

GF DF

I adore the flavours in this one. Salmon is a great source of omega-3s, healthy fats that are important at any age, but especially during the menopause. Many studies suggest that increasing your omega-3 intake can support your mood, in part because omega-3s might lower levels of inflammation in the body.

4 x 120g (4¼oz) salmon fillets
1–2 tbsp red curry paste
2 tsp olive oil
2 tbsp pumpkin seeds
   (pepitas)
1 tbsp gluten-free soy sauce
Salsa
1 cucumber, deseeded,
   finely chopped
1 small red onion,
   finely chopped
Seeds from 1 pomegranate
Juice of 1 lime
1 green finger chilli, finely
   chopped
Handful of coriander (cilantro)
   leaves, chopped (optional)

1 For the salsa, combine the cucumber, red onion, pomegranate seeds, lime juice, chilli and coriander, if using, in a bowl. Season with sea salt and freshly ground black pepper and set aside.

2 Meanwhile, coat the salmon fillets all over in the red curry paste. Heat the oil in a non-stick frying pan over a medium-high heat and fry the fish, skin-side down, for 3–4 minutes until golden and crisp, then turn and cook for 1 minute.

3 Add the pumpkin seeds and soy sauce to the pan. Cover and cook for 3 minutes until the fish is just cooked through. Serve with the salsa.

Tips

Swap the salmon for other white fish fillets, like sea bass, or small chicken breasts, prawns or tofu. And try peanuts or cashew nuts instead of the pumpkin seeds. Serve with your favourite whole grain – brown or red rice or quinoa. For a low-carb option, serve with some greens like steamed pak choi.

Tuscan bean stew

Serves 4–6
Ready in 40 minutes

VO GF

The one thing all nutritional experts agree on is that we need to be eating more plants. This doesn't mean becoming vegatarian, but including some meat-free meal options is a good idea. This is a classic Italian one-pot meal and the richness comes from the diversity of plants. Looking after your gut is an essential part of a healthy menopause, and this recipe does that for you.

2 tbsp olive oil
1 large red onion, finely sliced
2 celery sticks, finely sliced
1 bulb fennel, finely sliced
200g (7oz) cavolo nero, sliced
1 sprig of fresh rosemary, or
    1 tsp dried
750ml (3 cups) fresh
    vegetable or chicken stock/
    bone broth (see page 227)
    (or use a gluten-free
    low-sodium stock cube)
1 x 400g (14oz) tin white
    (butter or cannellini) or
    borlotti beans, drained and
    rinsed
40g (1½oz) vegetarian hard
    cheese or parmesan
    shavings, to serve
Extra virgin olive oil, to drizzle

1 Heat the olive oil in a flameproof casserole dish over a medium heat and gently fry the onion, celery and fennel for 10 minutes until lovely and golden and soft.

2 Add the cavolo nero, rosemary and stock and season with sea salt and freshly ground black pepper. Bring to the boil, then reduce to a simmer and cook gently for 10 minutes before adding the beans.

3 Simmer for a further 10 minutes, then serve in bowls with a scattering of cheese shavings and a drizzle of extra virgin olive oil.

Tips

Double up for easy batch-cooking and freeze in portions for up to a month (defrost fully before reheating). Enjoy with some sourdough bread.

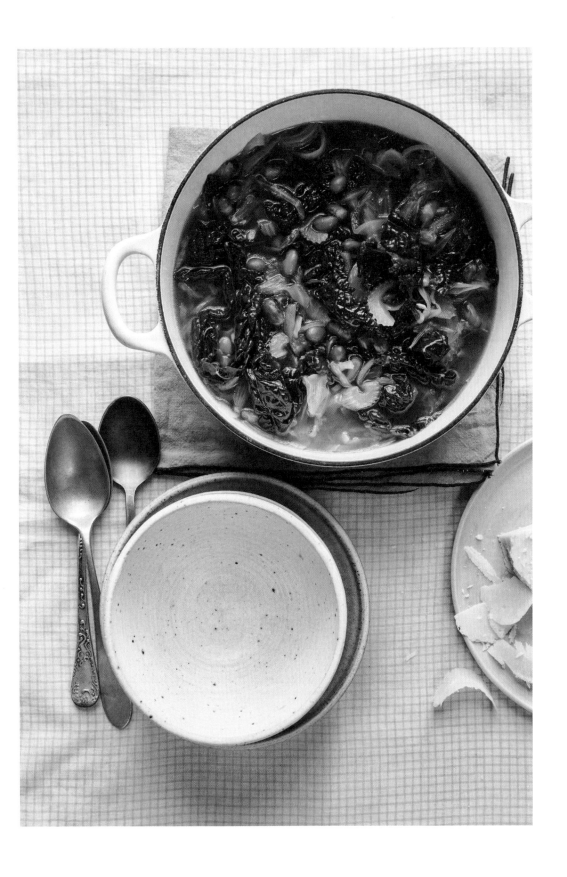

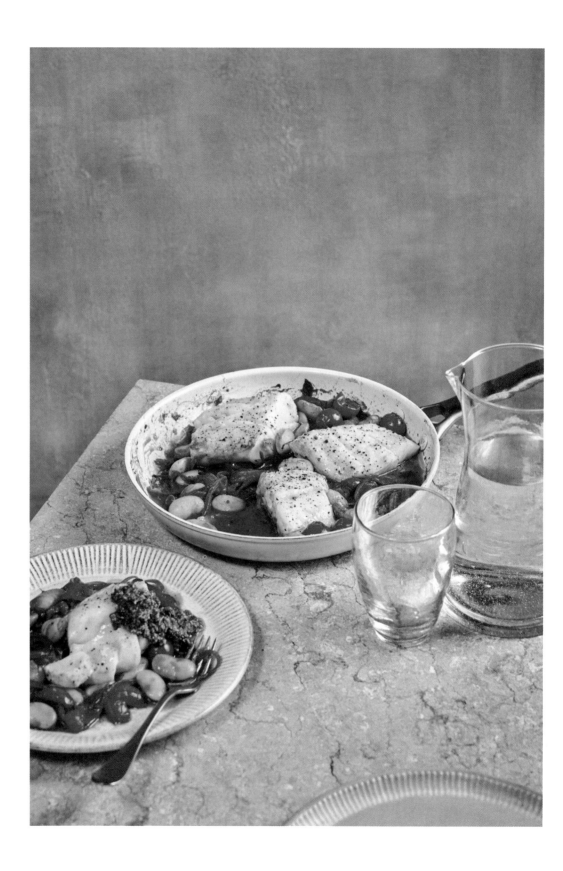

Cod with pumpkin-seed pesto

Serves 4
Ready in 40 minutes

GF

This is a wonderfully light and tasty dinner, but if you want the meal to be even lighter, you can take out the beans. Pumpkin seeds are the hero ingredient in this recipe. I love them, and it's amazing to think that such a little seed is such a nutrient powerhouse, so it's a good idea to incorporate them into your diet often. Pumpkin seeds are high in zinc, which is needed to keep your skin, hair and nails healthy, bones strong, libido up and immune system working for you – all important factors during the menopause.

2 tbsp Garlic oil (see page 224)
1 large red onion, sliced
1 x 400g (14oz) tin cherry tomatoes
190g (7oz) roasted red peppers (capsicums), sliced
1 x 400g (14oz) tin butter beans, drained and rinsed
1 tsp apple cider vinegar
4 x 150g (5½oz) cod fillets, or any white fish fillets

Pesto
3 tbsp pumpkin seeds (pepitas)
50g (2oz) wild rocket (arugula)
20g (½ cup) fresh basil leaves
1 clove garlic (optional)
30g (⅓ cup) grated vegetarian hard cheese or parmesan
3 tbsp extra virgin olive oil
Juice of ½ lemon

1 Preheat the oven to 180°C (350°F).

2 Heat the oil in an ovenproof frying pan over a medium heat and gently fry the onion for 5 minutes until softened. Add the cherry tomatoes and red pepper and cook for 10–12 minutes until the tomatoes start to break down into a lovely sauce. Add the butter beans and vinegar, season with sea salt and freshly ground black pepper and simmer for a few minutes more.

3 Nestle the cod fillets into the pan, cover and transfer to the oven to bake for 15 minutes until the fish is just cooked.

4 Meanwhile, make the pesto. Toast the pumpkin seeds in a dry pan over a low heat for 5 minutes until they burst, then tip into a small food processor along with the rocket, basil, garlic, if using, and cheese. Whizz together, drizzling in the olive oil until you have a thick, luscious pesto. Add lemon juice and 1–2 tablespoons water to loosen and season to taste. Serve with the cod.

Tips

Any leftover pesto will keep in the fridge for up to a week. It is delicious served with pasta, or you can mix it with some natural yoghurt and use it as a dip for crudités or breadsticks. You can serve this with the Turmeric-spiced sweet potato wedges on page 222.

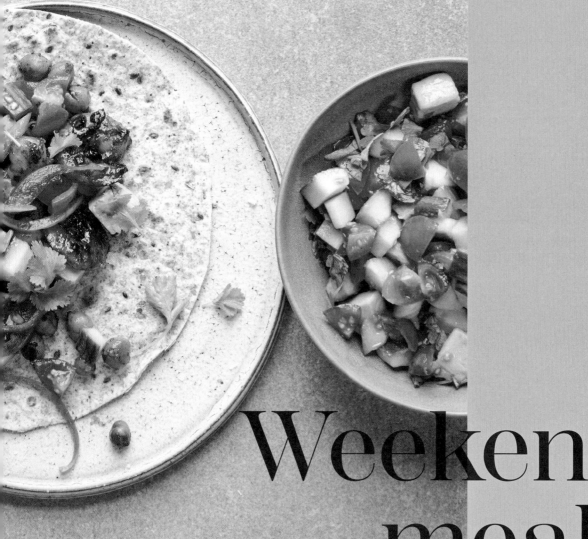

Weekend meals

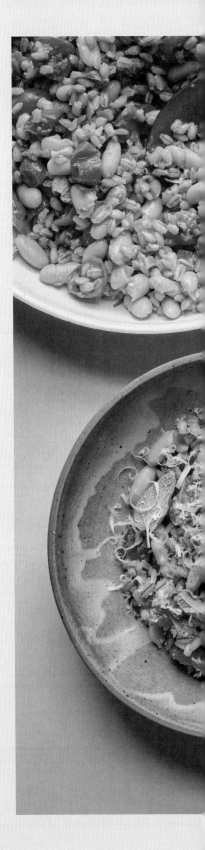

Healthy eating when you are trying to maintain your weight is about eating in balance 80 per cent of the time, and then including some of your favourite foods or meals that are more indulgent than normal 20 per cent of the time. The recipes in this chapter are a mixed bag. Some are well balanced and could easily be part of your 80 per cent, but just take longer to cook than the previous recipes. Others are more indulgent and are more your 20-per-cent-of-the-time meals. Being a dietitian, I'm always looking for ways to make recipes as nutritious as possible without losing out on the taste, so, even for meals that are more indulgent, I will add in some veggies or reduce the sugar as much as I possibly can.

Easy shakshuka
with spinach

Serves 4
Ready in 40 minutes

V GF

One of the things I look forward to the most on the weekend is a good brunch. This is my all-time favourite brunch meal. It's a simple combination of tomatoes, onions, spices and herbs with gently cooked eggs. Often, I make extra tomato sauce on the weekend, keep it in the fridge and then just heat it up and add the eggs on weekdays. This way, I can bring brunch yumminess into my week. Where I can, I always try to squeeze another vegetable into my recipes (in this case spinach) for even more plant diversity. Diverse diet = diverse microbiome = healthy hormones.

2 tbsp Garlic oil (see page 224)
1 large red onion, very finely sliced
2 red peppers (capsicums), deseeded and finely sliced
2 tsp cumin seeds
1 tsp hot smoked paprika
1 tsp sweet smoked paprika
2 x 400g (14oz) tins plum tomatoes
150g (5½oz) baby spinach
4 medium eggs
Large handful of fresh coriander (cilantro) (optional)
100g (⅓ cup) natural yoghurt
Sprinkling of sumac

1 Heat the oil in a large non-stick pan over a medium-low heat and gently fry the onion and pepper for 10 minutes. Add the spices and fry for 1 minute more, then add the tomatoes and break them up with the back of your spoon.

2 Season with sea salt and freshly ground black pepper and simmer gently for 15–20 minutes, then add the spinach and cook until the spinach has wilted down.

3 Make four hollows in the sauce and crack an egg into each, then cover and cook for 4–5 minutes until the whites are set but the yolks are still a bit runny.

4 Scatter with coriander, if using, and serve with dollops of yoghurt, a sprinkling of sumac and freshly ground black pepper.

Tips

If your eggs are not the freshest, you can drain any excess loose white by tipping them into a sieve and letting them drain for 30 seconds before cooking. Serve with crusty sourdough bread.

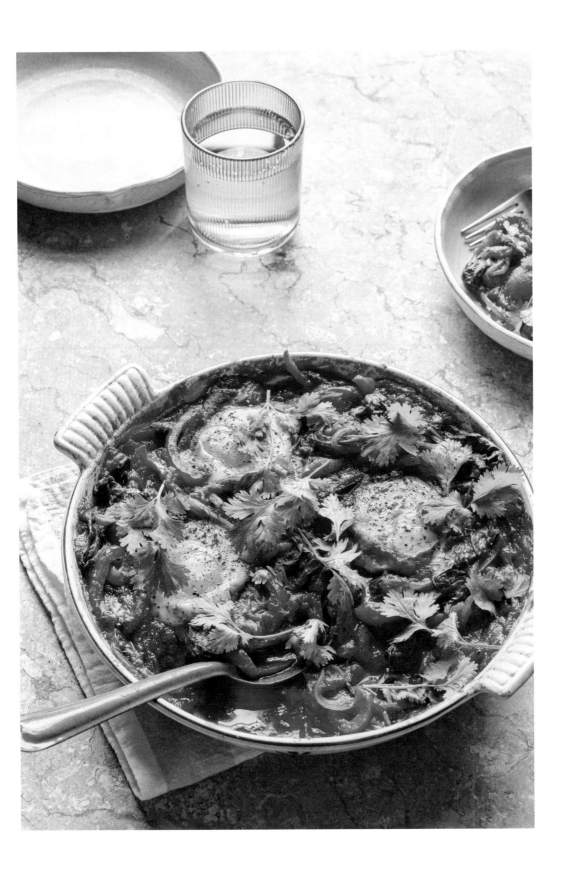

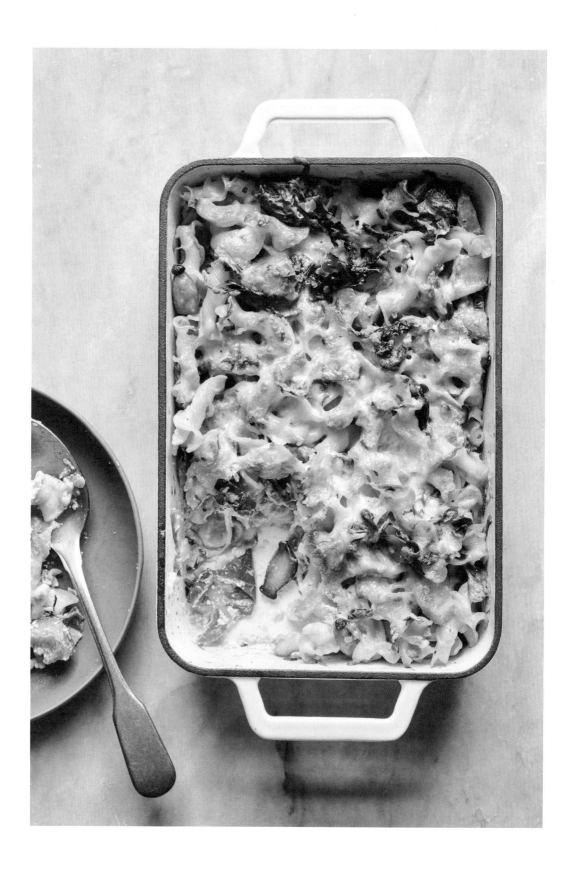

Mushroom and pumpkin pasta al forno

Serves 4-6
Ready in 1 hour

VO

350g (12oz) short pasta
3 tbsp olive oil
1 red onion, finely chopped
5–6 fresh sage leaves,
    finely chopped
1 tbsp plain (all-purpose) flour
350–400ml (scant 1½–1⅔
    cups) fresh vegetable stock
    (or use a low-sodium stock
    cube)
200g (7oz) mushrooms,
    finely chopped
300g (10½oz) pumpkin, peeled
    and diced
½ large Savoy cabbage,
    shredded, or 200g (7oz)
    baby spinach
150g (⅔ cup) soft ricotta
    cheese
100g (1 cup) grated cheddar,
    vegetarian hard cheese or
    parmesan (optional)
120g (1 cup) torn vegetarian
    mozzarella cheese

Virginia was my first 'Italian' friend when I moved to Milan. A mutual friend set us up and we hit it off straight away. Her family has since become '*la mia famaglia*', and I have enjoyed many looooonnng Italian-style Sunday lunches at her house. Pasta al forno is a firm favourite and an Italian classic. This recipe is based on Virginia's mum Patricia's recipe, although, of course, I have found a way to add in extra vegetables. This version is made with vegetables only, but you can also make it with a meat ragu or bolognese.

1 Bring a saucepan of salted water to the boil and cook the pasta for 8–10 minutes until al dente, but tender.

2 Meanwhile, heat half the olive oil in a pan over a medium heat and gently fry the onion and sage for 5 minutes. Add the flour and cook for 1-2 minutes, then gradually add the stock, stirring until you have a smooth sauce. Season with sea salt and freshly ground black pepper and simmer gently for 5 minutes.

3 Heat the rest of the oil in a second pan over a medium-high heat and fry the mushroom until golden. Add the pumpkin and cook for 4–5 minutes until the pumpkin is starting to become tender. Add the cabbage or spinach and allow to wilt for a minute or two.

4 Preheat the oven to 200°C (400°F).

5 Combine the sauce with the vegetables and stir in the ricotta and most of the cheddar or parmesan, if using.

6 Drain the pasta, reserving a cup of the cooking water. Toss the pasta with the sauce, adding enough water to loosen if needed. Spoon into an ovenproof dish.

7 Scatter with the remaining cheddar or parmesan and the mozzarella and bake for 30 minutes until golden and bubbling.

Tip

You can freeze this for up to 3 months (defrost fully before reheating).

Italian-style roasted sea bass with potatoes

Serves 4
Ready in 1 hour

GF DF

Coming to my house for dinner? There's a good chance I will serve you this. It's simple, it's delicious and this one is healthy. I go all out and make an occasion of going to the fishmonger and choosing my fish. It may look like a complicated dish, but it really isn't, and during the week I also make it using fish fillets for a healthy and easy dinner. In general, we don't eat enough fish. By simply eating one portion of fish a week, you'll live longer!

350g (12oz) new potatoes, thickly sliced
400g (2⅓ cups) cherry tomatoes
1 red onion, cut into wedges
2 tbsp olive oil
Good pinch of chilli flakes
4 anchovies, chopped
2 tbsp capers
1 whole sea bass, cleaned (about 1kg/2lb 4oz)
1 lemon, sliced
Handful of fresh basil leaves
Handful of fresh flat-leaf parsley

1 Preheat the oven to 190°C (375°F).

2 Tumble the potato into a roasting tin with the cherry tomatoes and red onion. Drizzle with the oil, scatter over the chilli flakes and roast for 25–30 minutes until the potato is tender to the point of a knife and turning golden.

3 Toss in the anchovy and capers, then lay the sea bass on top. Stuff some of the lemon into the cavity, along with half the herbs. Arrange the rest of the lemon around the fish. Season with sea salt and freshly ground black pepper and roast for 20 minutes until the fish is cooked through.

4 Spoon the juicy tomatoes over the fish and serve scattered with the remaining herbs.

Tip

You can use this same recipe for a sausage bake instead of sea bass. Just leave out the lemon slices and bake for 30-35 minutes.

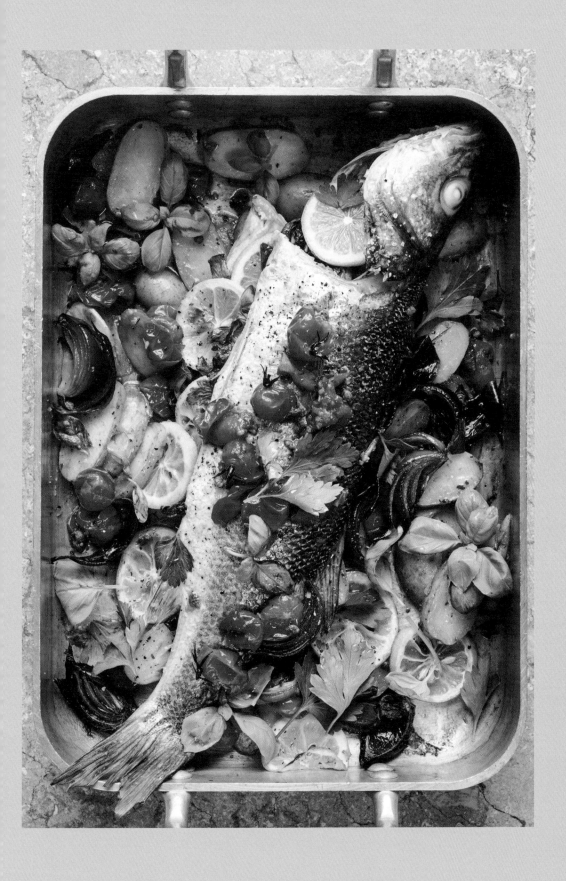

Mix-it-up cottage pie

Serves 6
Ready in 1 hour 20 minutes

GF

2 tbsp olive oil or Garlic oil
  (see page 224)
1 red onion, finely sliced
1 carrot, finely diced
2 celery sticks, finely chopped
100g (3½oz) button
  mushrooms, very finely
  chopped
500g (1lb 2 oz) beef mince
60g (generous ¼ cup) green
  or brown lentils
2 tbsp tomato paste
  (concentrated purée)
2 tbsp gluten-free
  Worcestershire sauce
300ml (1¼ cups) fresh beef
  stock or Chicken bone broth
  (see page 227) (or use a
  gluten-free low-sodium
  stock cube)
2 bay leaves (fresh or dried)
4 sprigs of fresh thyme or
  ½ tsp ground
Mash
500g (1lb 2oz) floury potatoes,
  peeled
300g (10½oz) sweet potatoes
  or butternut squash, peeled
2 parsnips, peeled
Splash of milk or plant milk
  of choice
60g (⅔ cup) grated cheddar
  cheese (optional)

A classic family favourite with the twist of added lentils, mushrooms and an array of root veggies to make it more Mediterranean. Prep this in advance and freeze, and you'll have a brilliantly balanced and nutritious meal ready for busy days. You just need to add some greens and you're good to go. Using sweet potato or pumpkin for the top of the pie not only adds sweetness but also provides you with more antioxidants, which work on a cellular level to keep your body out of oxidative stress.

1 Heat the oil in a large frying pan over a medium heat and gently fry the onion, carrot and celery for 10 minutes until lovely and soft.

2 Add the mushroom, increase the heat to medium-high and fry for a further 5–10 minutes until golden.

3 Add the mince and increase the heat to high. Brown all over, breaking up the mince with your spoon. Add the lentils, tomato paste, Worcestershire sauce and stock. Season to taste.

4 Add the herbs and bring to the boil, then reduce the heat and simmer for 20–25 minutes until the sauce is thick and reduced and the lentils are tender.

5 Meanwhile, to make the mash, chop the vegetables into even-sized pieces and place in a large pan of cold, salted water. Bring to the boil and simmer gently for 20 minutes. Drain and return to the pan over a low heat. Add the milk and season, then mash with a potato masher.

6 Preheat the oven to 200°C (400°F).

7 Spoon the sauce into a 1.2 litre (42fl oz) ovenproof dish. Top with the mash, scatter over the cheddar, if using, and bake for 30–35 minutes until golden and bubbling.

Tips

You can double this up easily to batch-cook. Freeze, unbaked, for up to 3 months. Add 20 minutes to the cooking time to cook from frozen.

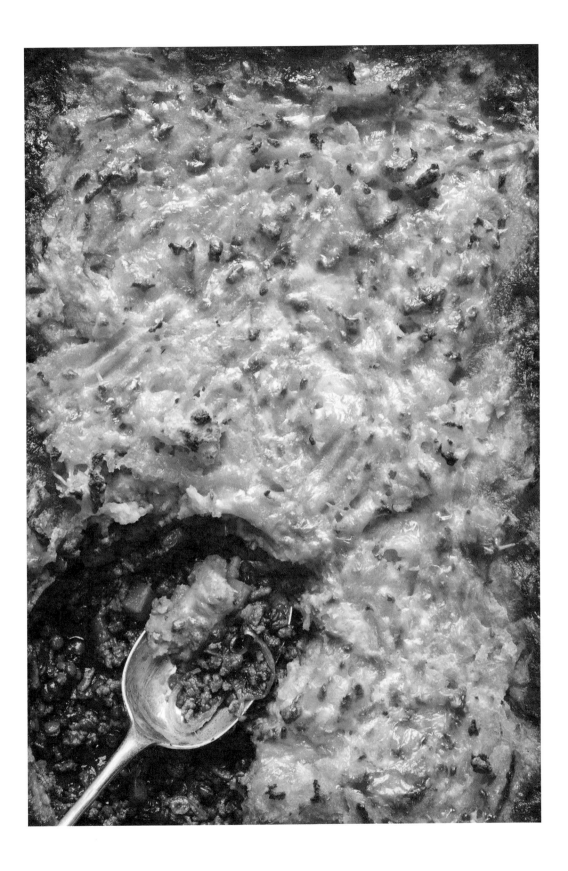

Red bean and aubergine ragu

Serves 8
Ready in 1½ hours

VO GF

A comforting and delicious plant-based meal that is flavourful and packed with nutrients and plant diversity. During the menopause, you need to prioritise looking after your gut microbiome. This means eating a diverse range of plant-based foods every day. You should be aiming for 30 points per week (see page 67), and this recipe gives you about 8 points.

3 tbsp olive oil
1 onion, finely chopped
2 aubergines (eggplants), diced into 1cm (½ inch) pieces
2 celery sticks, finely chopped
1 large carrot, finely chopped
2 tsp fennel seeds
Good pinch of chilli flakes
200ml (generous ¾ cup) white wine (optional)
2 x 400g (14oz) tins plum tomatoes
200ml (generous ¾ cup) fresh vegetable stock (or use a gluten-free low-sodium stock cube)
2 x 400g (14oz) tins red kidney beans, drained and rinsed
25g (¼ cup) grated vegetarian hard cheese or parmesan

1 Heat the olive oil in a large non-stick frying pan over a medium-low heat and gently fry the onion, aubergine, celery, carrot, fennel seeds and chilli flakes for 20 minutes until very soft and golden.

2 Add the white wine, if using, and bubble for 3–4 minutes, then stir in the tomatoes. Break up the tomatoes with the back of your spoon, then season well with sea salt and freshly ground black pepper.

3 Add the vegetable stock and bring to the boil, then reduce the heat and simmer gently for 30 minutes, adding a splash of water if it starts to reduce too far.

4 Add the kidney beans and simmer for 10-15 minutes more, then serve with the grated cheese.

Tips

This freezes brilliantly for up to 3 months (defrost fully before reheating). You can serve with brown rice or, for a lower-carb option, steamed vegetables.

Black bean and sweet potato tacos

Serves 4
Ready in 45 minutes

V

When I share recipe ideas with my clients, I often get asked for some good healthy taco recipes! Well, here you go. This option is vegetarian. Black beans, like other legumes, are prized for their high protein and fibre content. And not only do they add a vibrant colour to the recipe and give your body an antioxidant boost, they are also a good plant-based source of calcium, helping to support healthy bones.

4 medium sweet potatoes (about 650g/1lb 7oz), diced
2 tbsp olive oil
2 tsp ground cumin
1 tsp sweet smoked paprika
½ tsp dried oregano
1 x 400g (14oz) tin black beans, drained and rinsed
½ red cabbage, finely sliced
Juice of 1 lime, plus extra, to serve
150g (¾ cup) cooked sweetcorn
4 large or 8 small flour tortillas (see page 226)
Handful of fresh coriander (cilantro), roughly chopped (optional)
80g (¾ cup) grated cheddar cheese (optional)
4 tbsp natural yoghurt

1 Preheat the oven to 200°C (400°F).

2 Toss the sweet potato in a roasting tin with the olive oil, spices and oregano. Roast for 30 minutes, turning once. Add the black beans and roast for a further 5 minutes.

3 Meanwhile, toss the red cabbage in a bowl with the lime juice and sweetcorn and season with a little sea salt and freshly ground black pepper.

4 Warm the tortillas in a dry frying pan and serve with the sweet potato and black beans, the red cabbage slaw and some chopped coriander, if using. Add a scattering of cheese, if using, and a dollop of yoghurt and serve.

HELPS WITH | strong bones | healthy skin

Tip

If you don't have time to make homemade tortillas, you can use some shop-bought alternatives.

Sticky caramelised prawn tacos

Serves 4
Ready in 20 minutes

My five-year-old nephew, who is the fussiest of eaters, gave these the thumbs-up, which means they must be good! Adding the chickpeas gives you about 20 per cent of your fibre intake for the day. Prawns are often demonised for being high in cholesterol. However, dietary cholesterol doesn't push up your cholesterol numbers the way we once thought. Too much saturated fat and sugar does. Prawns are rich in protein and are a useful source of the B group of vitamins – important vitamins for energy production.

1 red onion, finely sliced
2 limes
1 tbsp Garlic oil (see page 224)
350g (12oz) raw prawns
1 x 400g (14oz) tin chickpeas, drained and rinsed
2 tsp chipotle paste
2 tsp honey
½ large cucumber, deseeded and diced
150g (1 cup) cherry tomatoes, diced
1 ripe avocado, diced
Small handful of fresh coriander (cilantro) (optional)
4 large or 8 small flour tortillas (see page 226)
4 tbsp natural yoghurt (optional)

1 In a bowl, toss the red onion with the juice of 1 lime and a little sea salt and set aside.

2 Heat a non-stick frying pan over a medium-high heat. Add the garlic oil and prawns and fry for 2–3 minutes until the prawns are just turning pink all over. Add the chickpeas and cook for a minute more, then add the chipotle paste and honey and cook for 1–2 minutes until sticky.

3 Combine the cucumber, tomato, avocado and coriander, if using, with the red onion. Check the seasoning.

4 Warm the tortillas in a dry frying pan and serve with the prawns, salsa and a dollop of yoghurt, if using. Cut the remaining lime into wedges to squeeze over.

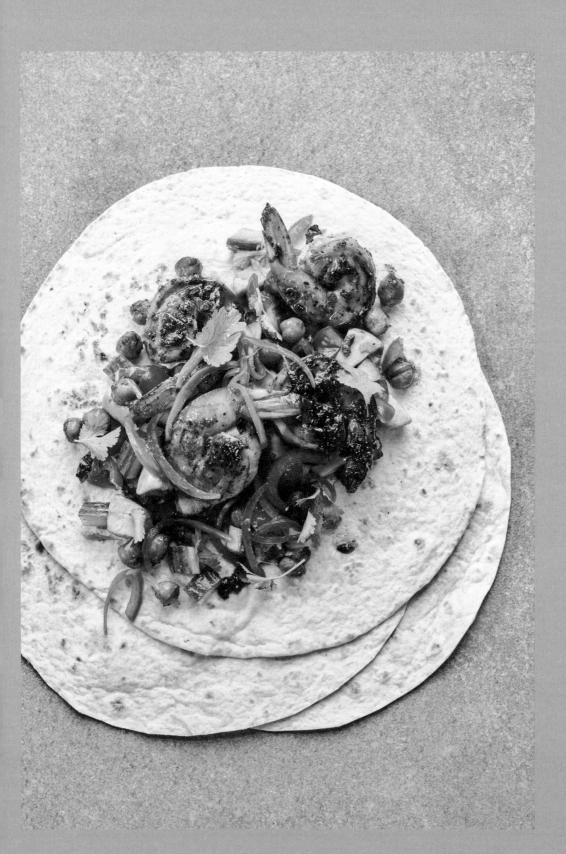

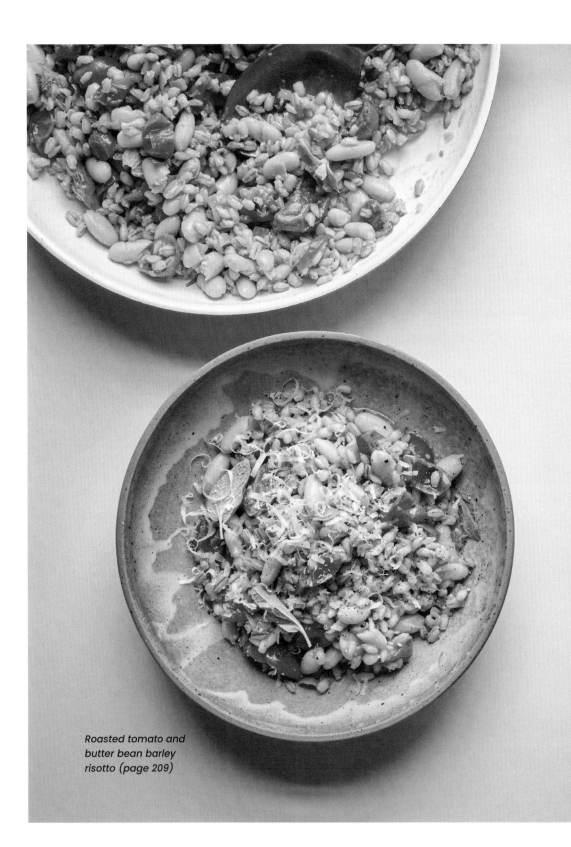

Roasted tomato and butter bean barley risotto (page 209)

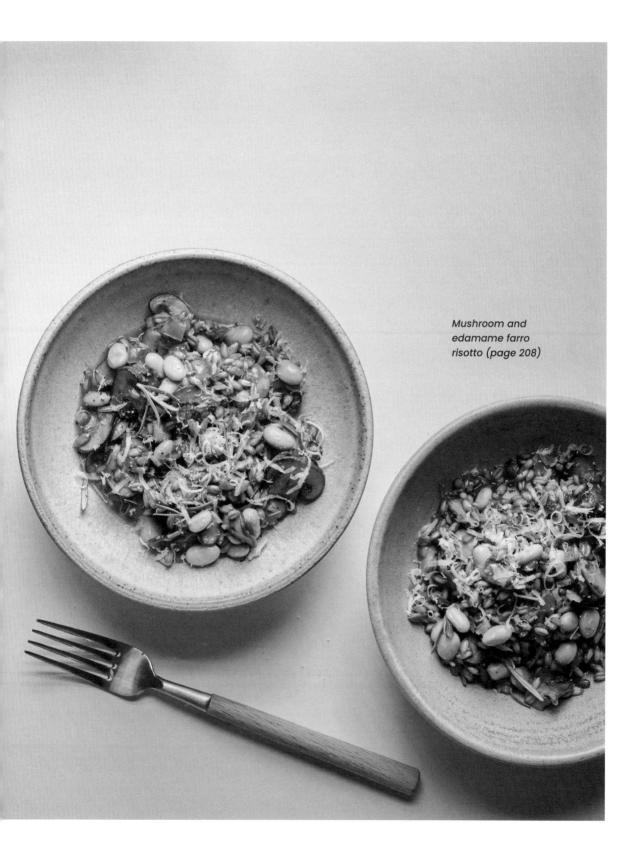

Mushroom and edamame farro risotto (page 208)

Mushroom and edamame farro risotto

Serves 4-6
Ready in 1 hour 10 minutes

VO

Risottos typically contain arborio rice, which is a short-grain rice with a high starch content and a high glycaemic index. It's not great for blood-glucose levels. This recipe uses farro, which is an ancient whole grain that works brilliantly in risottos and is much better for your blood-sugar levels. Adding the edamame and mushrooms also boosts the protein content to about 12 grams per portion. To give it even more of a boost, toss in a handful of pumpkin seeds (pepitas) before serving.

3 tbsp olive oil
1 red onion, finely chopped
300g (10½oz) chestnut
 mushrooms, finely sliced
250g (9oz) farro grains
125ml (½ cup) white wine
 (optional)
750ml (3 cups) fresh
 vegetable or chicken stock
 or Chicken bone broth (see
 page 227) (or use 2 low-
 sodium stock cubes)
1 sprig of fresh rosemary,
 needles stripped or ½ tsp
 dried
Small knob of butter
125g (4½oz) frozen edamame
 beans, defrosted
50g (½ cup) grated
 vegetarian hard cheese or
 parmesan

1 Heat the olive oil in a sauté pan over a medium heat and fry the onion and mushroom for 10 minutes until the onion is softened and the mushroom is golden. Add the farro and toast for a couple of minutes.

2 Add the wine, if using, and bubble away for 2–3 minutes. Pour in the stock, add the rosemary and season with sea salt and freshly ground black pepper. Simmer gently, stirring every so often, for 35–40 minutes until most of the stock has been absorbed but it is still juicy.

3 Add the knob of butter, the edamame and cheese, then remove from the heat, cover and leave to stand for 5 minutes before serving.

Tips

If you can't get farro, try spelt. The grains will be a little firmer but still delicious.

Roasted tomato and butter bean barley risotto

Serves 4
Ready in 1 hour 10 minutes

VO

This is a super-tasty risotto. Risottos are typically low in protein, but during the menopause you need to ensure that each meal contains some protein to optimise your blood-glucose control and protect your precious muscle mass. I added butter beans to this recipe to give the risotto a boost in protein and, of course, fibre.

300g (2 cups) cherry tomatoes, halved
3 tbsp olive oil
4 sprigs of fresh oregano, leaves stripped, or 1 tsp dried
1 red onion, finely chopped
250g (1¼ cups) pearl barley
800ml (3¼ cups) fresh vegetable or chicken stock or Chicken bone broth (see page 227) (or use 2 low-sodium stock cubes)
1 x 400g (14oz) tin butter beans, drained and rinsed
200g (7oz) cavolo nero, finely shredded (optional)
60g (⅔ cup) grated vegetarian hard cheese or parmesan
Handful of fresh basil leaves, to serve

1 Preheat the oven to 180°C (350°F).

2 Put the tomato into a roasting tin, drizzle with half the olive oil and scatter with the oregano. Season well with sea salt and freshly ground black pepper and roast for 40–50 minutes until sticky and golden.

3 Meanwhile, heat the rest of the oil in a sauté pan over a medium heat and fry the onion for 5 minutes until softened. Add the pearly barley and stock, season and simmer for 40–45 minutes until almost all the stock has been absorbed and the grains are tender.

4 Add the tomato, butter beans, cavolo nero, if using, and a good splash of water. Cover and cook gently for 3–4 minutes.

5 Stir in the cheese and set aside to rest, covered, for 5 minutes before scattering with basil leaves and serving.

gut health | blood-glucose control

HELPS WITH

Tip

Other great flavours to try in a pearl barley risotto would be roasted butternut squash and sage or asparagus and peas with mint.

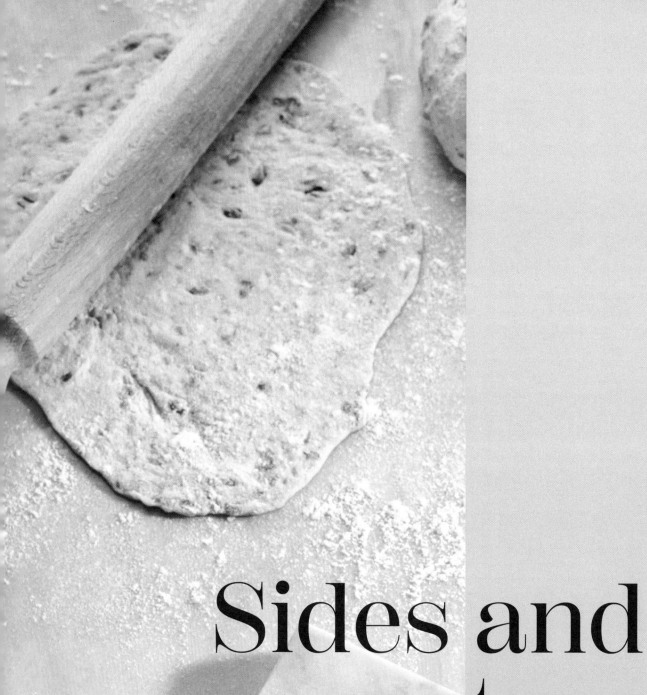

Sides and extras

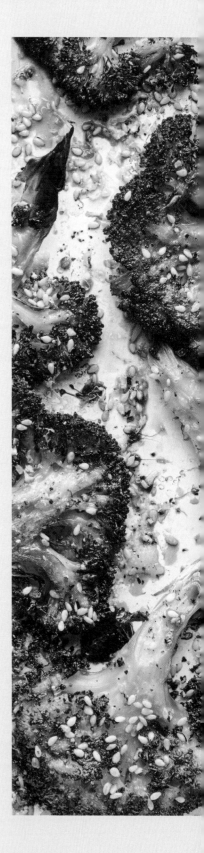

I often ask my clients to eat more vegetables and they frequently ask me for inspiration on different ways to prepare them. Vegetables don't have to be boring! In this section, you will find some of my favourite ways to prepare vegetables. Mix and match within the recipes, as variety is the spice of life. I've also included some of my go-to extra recipes. I love the flavour of garlic, for example, but garlic makes me, and many women with sensitive guts, bloat. Garlic oil gives you the flavour without the bloat. Flatbreads and tortillas are a great addition to any main meal. And while I cannot make bold scientific claims about the benefits of broths, they feel utterly nourishing and are good for the soul, so I've included a chicken bone broth here.

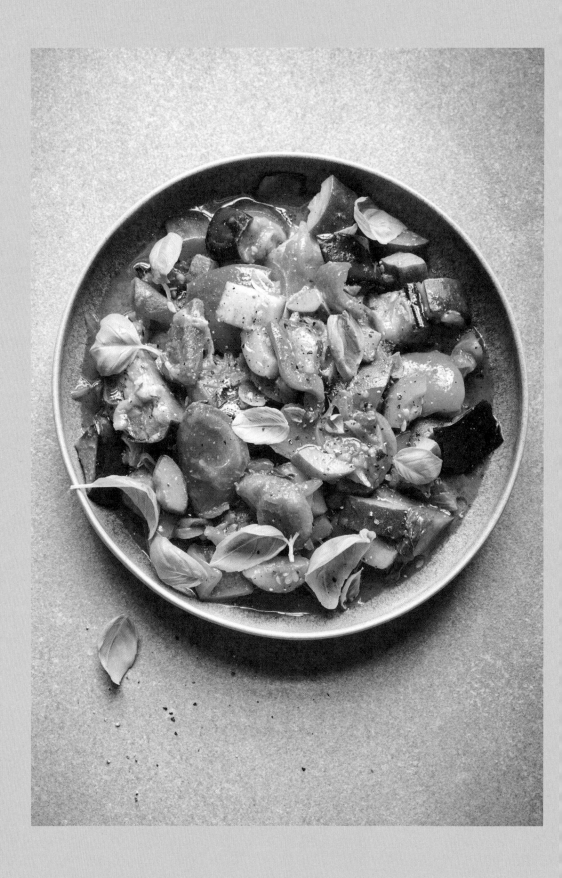

Classic ratatouille

Serves 6
Ready in 55 minutes

VG GF

This super-healthy traditional French recipe is a brilliant way to get in your plant diversity, and it can be eaten as a side for lunch or dinner. The diversity in the number of plants will rack up your plant points (see page 67). You need to aim for thirty different plants for the week – you have at least 9 points here!

100ml (scant ½ cup) olive oil
1 aubergine (eggplant), diced
1 red onion, finely sliced
3 courgettes (zucchini), diced
2 red peppers (capsicums),
    deseeded and diced
500g (1lb 2oz) large ripe
    tomatoes, chopped
1 bulb garlic, cloves separated
    and peeled
4-5 sprigs of fresh thyme,
    leaves picked
Bunch of fresh basil
Good pinch of chilli flakes
100ml (scant ½ cup) water

1 Heat the olive oil in a large casserole dish over a medium-low heat and fry the aubergine for 10–12 minutes until it is golden and tender and has started to release the oil back into the pan. Scoop out of the dish and set aside. You can remove all but 2 tablespoons of the oil at this point.

2 Add the onion, courgette and pepper to the pan and fry for 10 minutes until lovely and softened.

3 Return the aubergine to the pan along with the tomato, garlic, thyme, most of the basil and a good pinch of chilli flakes. Season with sea salt and freshly ground black pepper, add the water and cook, covered, for 20–25 minutes.

4 Check the seasoning, remove the garlic cloves and serve topped with extra fresh basil.

Tips

For an autumnal ratatouille, substitute the courgette and aubergine for pumpkin and use tinned tomatoes. You can also add a tin of chickpeas and some paprika for a Spanish twist. This would be fabulous on its own or stirred through pasta. It would also be a great accompaniment to grilled chicken or pan-fried cod. If you would prefer not to use garlic, use Garlic oil (page 224) instead of olive oil.

Garlic, lemon and chilli sprouts

Serves 4
Ready in 35 minutes

V   GF   DF

500g (1lb 2oz) brussels
    sprouts
2 tbsp Garlic oil (see
    page 224)
1 red chilli, finely sliced, or
    pinch of chilli flakes
Finely grated zest of 1 lemon
30g (⅓ cup) flaked almonds

I am all about the nutritional extras you can add to your meals, and the flaked almonds on top are your extra here. They provide healthy fats for your skin and heart.

1 Preheat the oven to 200°C (400°F).

2 Blanch the sprouts in boiling water for 2-3 minutes, then drain and cut in half.

3 Tumble into a roasting tin and toss with the garlic oil, chilli and lemon zest. Season with sea salt and freshly ground black pepper. Arrange the brussels sprouts so they are cut-side down. Roast for 20 minutes, then scatter with the flaked almonds, toss together and roast for 5 minutes more. Serve.

Roasted red cabbage

Serves 4–6
Ready in 50 minutes

V   GF   DF

1 red cabbage, cut into
    wedges
1 tbsp olive oil
1 tsp fennel seeds
1 tbsp honey
2 oranges
1 tbsp balsamic vinegar
3 tbsp extra virgin olive oil
30g (¼ cup) pine nuts, toasted

I use red cabbage a lot in my cooking as it's rich in powerful antioxidants called anthocyanins, as well as a spectrum of nutrients, so it's the perfect addition for radiant skin. However, you can use any type of cabbage here.

1 Preheat the oven to 200°C (400°F).

2 Put the cabbage into a roasting tin, drizzle with the oil, sprinkle with fennel seeds and season with sea salt and freshly ground black pepper. Roast for 25 minutes, then turn and drizzle with the honey and roast for a further 10 minutes.

3 Meanwhile, segment the oranges, saving the juice in a bowl. Whisk the juice with the vinegar and extra virgin olive oil. Season.

4 Arrange cabbage on a platter. Cool to room temperature, then toss with the orange and pine nuts and drizzle with the dressing.

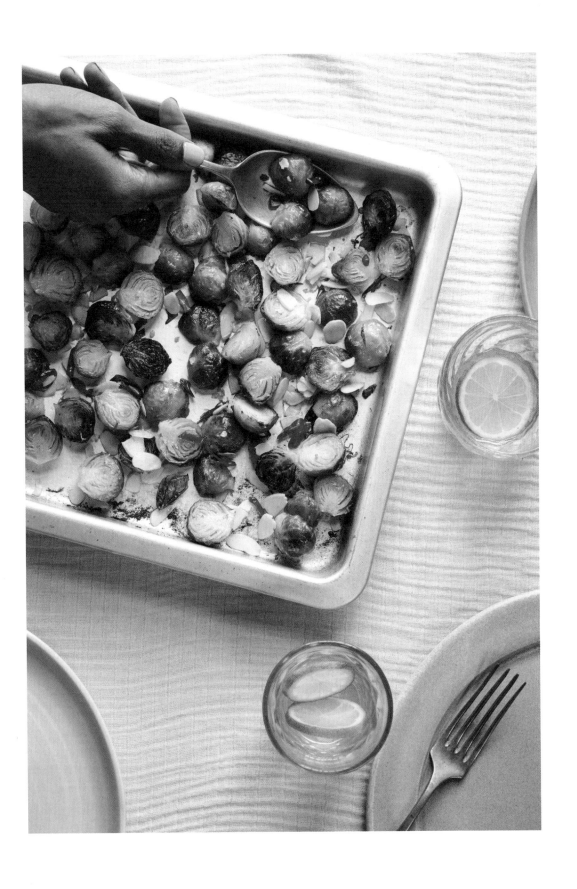

Red cabbage slaw with tahini dressing

Serves 4–6 as a side
Ready in 15 minutes

V GF

A simple red cabbage slaw that is easy and mayo-free, meaning it's much healthier! It's full of flavour and bursting with nutritional goodness too. The hero ingredients are the sesame seeds and tahini (sesame paste). Sesame seeds are small but mighty. They are one of the best plant-based sources of both calcium and iron and also contain magnesium and B vitamins. All these nutrients are on a menopausal woman's hit list for strong bones, better mood and more energy.

½ large red cabbage
2 large carrots
2 celery sticks
1 large apple
2 spring onions (scallions)
1 punnet of mustard cress
   (optional)
1 tbsp sesame seeds, toasted
Dressing
2 tbsp tahini
2 tbsp apple cider vinegar
2 tsp honey
75g (¼ cup) natural yoghurt
2 tbsp extra virgin olive oil

1 Very finely shred the cabbage and put into a large bowl. Julienne (or coarsely grate) the carrot, finely slice the celery and add both to the bowl.

2 Grate the apple, including the skin, with a box grater and add to the bowl. Finely slice the spring onions, snip the tops from the cress and toss both through the mixture.

3 In a bowl, whisk all the ingredients for the dressing, then pour over the slaw. Toss well, scatter with the seeds and serve.

Tips

If you have a mandolin, use it to shred the cabbage and slice the celery. You can play around with the ingredients here, too: try white cabbage instead of red, and a finely sliced firm green pear or peach instead of the apple. You can also try sprouting your own mung beans or lentils and adding them into the slaw instead of the cress.

Green beans with anchovies and tomatoes

Serves 4
Ready in 20 minutes

GF DF

I adore this combo – it bursts with flavour. Anchovies are a good source of omega-3, protein and vitamins. They are high in salt, so balancing them out with veggies like green beans, which are a good source of potassium, helps to negate the effects. Even in small servings, anchovies deliver calcium and selenium – key nutrients for your bones, skin and nails.

2 tbsp olive oil
1 clove garlic, whole, peeled (or use Garlic oil, see page 224)
3 anchovies
200g (7oz) tomatoes, roughly chopped
200g (7oz) green beans, trimmed
Handful of fresh basil leaves (optional)
Extra virgin olive oil, to drizzle

1 Heat the olive oil in a pan over a medium heat. Add the garlic and anchovies and fry for a minute until the anchovies have melted into the oil. Add the tomato, reduce the heat to low and cook for 10 minutes until broken down into a lovely thick sauce. Season to taste with sea salt and freshly ground black pepper and remove the garlic clove.

2 Meanwhile, blanch or steam the beans for 3–4 minutes until tender. Drain, reserving a splash of the water. Combine with the tomato sauce and add a little cooking water, if needed, to loosen.

3 Serve topped with the basil leaves, a drizzle of extra virgin olive oil and lots of black pepper.

HELPS WITH

Tip

This tomato sauce would also be delicious tossed through freshly cooked spaghetti.

Smashed broccoli

Serves 4
Ready in 35 minutes

VO GF

A smashing way to have your broccoli or even your cauliflower. The family will love this too. It goes well with any protein you may have – fish, chicken or plant-based options like tofu. Cruciferous veggies like broccoli are important additions to the menopause diet as they support the liver to metabolise oestrogens more efficiently. The sesame seeds are added to give you an extra calcium boost for your bones.

*1 large head of broccoli,
broken into florets or 300g
(10½oz) purple sprouting or
Tenderstem broccoli
(broccolini), trimmed*
2 tbsp olive oil
*20g (¼ cup) grated vegetarian
hard cheese or parmesan*
1 tbsp sesame seeds
1 tbsp gluten-free soy sauce

1 Preheat the oven to 210°C (410°F).

2 Blanch or steam the broccoli for 2–3 minutes. Drain, pat dry with kitchen towel and spread out on a baking sheet. Use the bottom of a glass to smash the florets so they are flattened but not mushed.

3 Drizzle with the olive oil and scatter with the cheese and sesame seeds. Season with black pepper and roast for 20–25 minutes until golden and crispy.

4 Drizzle with the soy sauce and serve.

Tip

You can also try this with cauliflower florets.

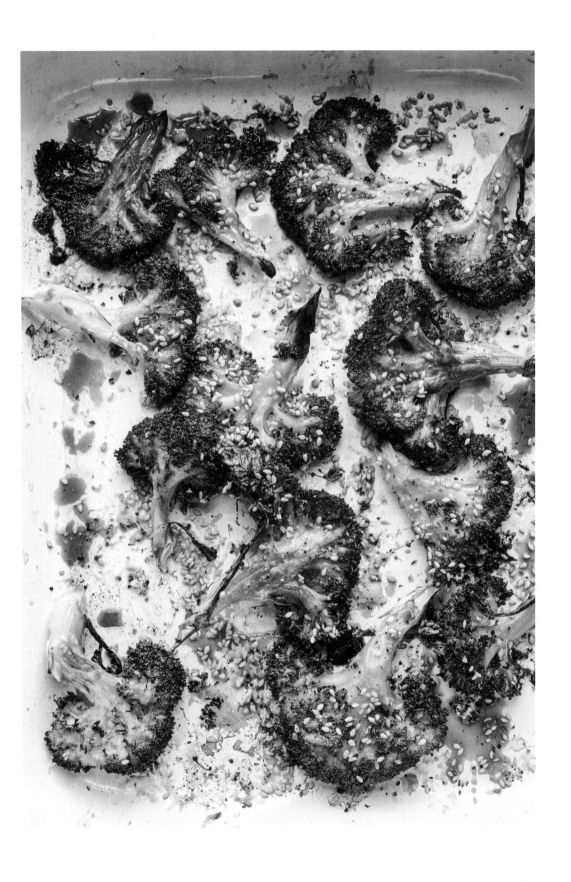

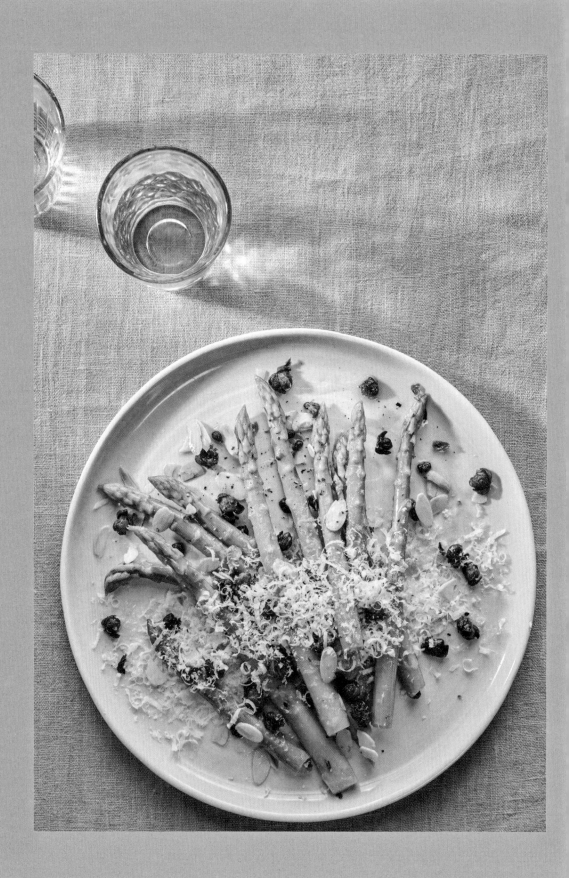

Asparagus with almonds and lemon

Serves 4
Ready in 15 minutes

VO GF

This is a nice fresh way of having your veggies. It works for pretty much every veggie, and I love it with green beans as well. Using extra virgin olive oil on your veggies to give them more flavour is so Mediterranean. The oil is a source of healthy fats and has some anti-inflammatory properties, but it is still a fat, so try not to overdo the portions!

250g (9oz) asparagus, trimmed
1 tbsp extra virgin olive oil, plus extra for drizzling
2 tbsp capers, drained and patted dry
Finely grated zest of 1 lemon
20g (¼ cup) grated vegetarian hard cheese or parmesan
20g (¼ cup) flaked almonds, toasted

1 Blanch or steam the asparagus for 2–3 minutes until tender to the point of a knife.

2 Heat the oil in a pan over a medium-high heat and add the capers. Cook for a couple of minutes until crispy. Reduce the heat to medium, add the asparagus and lemon zest and toss together. Season to taste with sea salt and freshly ground black pepper.

3 Arrange on a platter, scatter over the cheese and almonds and drizzle with extra virgin olive oil, if needed.

Tip

For a real treat, fry up some cured chorizo and toss through to make this a meal in itself.

Turmeric-spiced sweet potato wedges

Serves 4
Ready in 40 minutes

VG GF

Sweet potato wedges always remind me of eating out. However, you can easily make them at home and they taste just as good. I'm adding the super-spice turmeric here for its anti-inflammatory effects. You need to have a lot of turmeric to really get these effects. This isn't about going out there and buying high-dose supplements, but more about adding it regularly to your diet.

750g (1lb 10oz) sweet potatoes (unpeeled), cut into thin wedges
½ tsp ground turmeric
1 tsp ground coriander
Good pinch of cayenne pepper
2 tbsp olive oil
1 tbsp sesame seeds

1 Preheat the oven to 200°C (400°F).

2 In a roasting tray, toss the sweet potato together with the spices and olive oil. Season with sea salt and freshly ground black pepper and roast for 25 minutes. Turn, scatter with the sesame seeds and roast for a further 10 minutes until golden and crispy. Serve.

Tip

Great as a side dish for roast chicken or pan-fried fish.

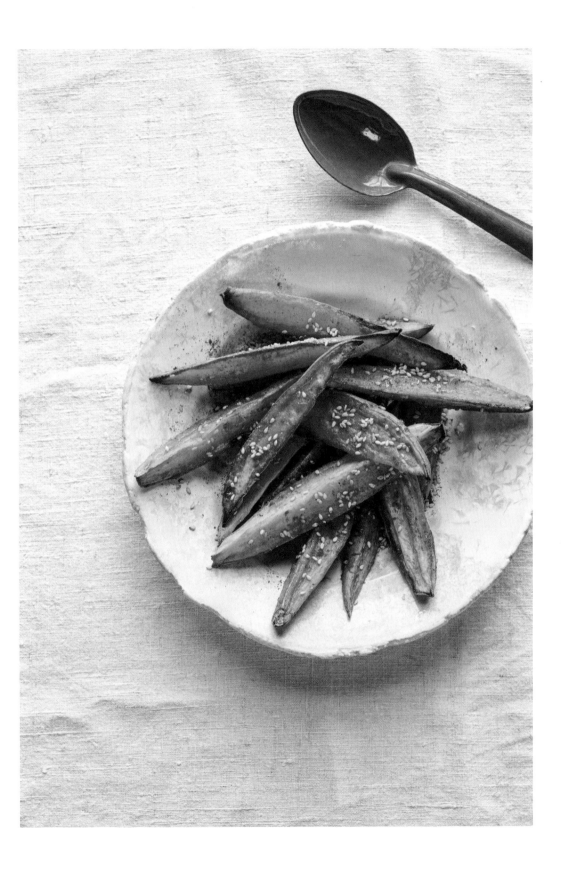

Garlic oil

bloating

HELPS WITH

Makes 500ml (17fl oz)
Ready in 15 minutes, plus
infusing time

VG GF

500ml (2 cups) olive oil or
  extra virgin olive oil
1 bulb of fresh garlic, peeled

Digestive issues, especially bloating, are a common symptom many women complain about. Garlic is high in FODMAPs, which are carbohydrates that can be difficult for some people, especially those with irritable bowels, to absorb. Including whole garlic in the diet can therefore cause bloating. However, garlic oil is low in FODMAPs, so you can have the flavour minus the bloat.

1 Gently warm the oil and garlic in a stainless-steel pan. You want it to be just warm and not boiling.

2 Remove from the heat and leave to infuse for a couple of hours, then strain into a sterilised jar or bottle.

Tips ——————————————————

If you like a stronger garlic flavour, you can halve the cloves before infusing. The oil will keep for up to a month (not in the fridge).

Simple flatbreads

gut health

HELPS WITH

Makes 8 flatbreads
Ready in 1½ hours

VG

400g (2½ cups) strong bread
  flour with seeds, plus extra,
  for dusting
1 tsp instant yeast
230ml (scant 1 cup) lukewarm
  water
4g (⅛oz) fine sea salt
2 tsp extra virgin olive oil,
  plus extra, for greasing

Every time I make a flatbread, I wonder why I buy them. They are simple to make, taste fantastic and don't contain a long list of preservatives and emulsifiers that aren't great for your gut microbiome. If you can't find a flour with seeds, add your own.

1 Put 50g (⅓ cup) of the flour into a bowl with the yeast and water and stand for 10 minutes. Add the rest of the flour, salt and oil. Turn out onto a lightly floured surface and knead well for 10 minutes, then transfer to an oiled bowl to rest in a warm place for 1 hour or until doubled in size.

2 Divide into eight portions and roll out into 20–25cm (8–10-inch) pieces.

3 Heat a heavy-based pan over a medium heat. Fry the breads in batches for 3–4 minutes each side until golden and puffed.

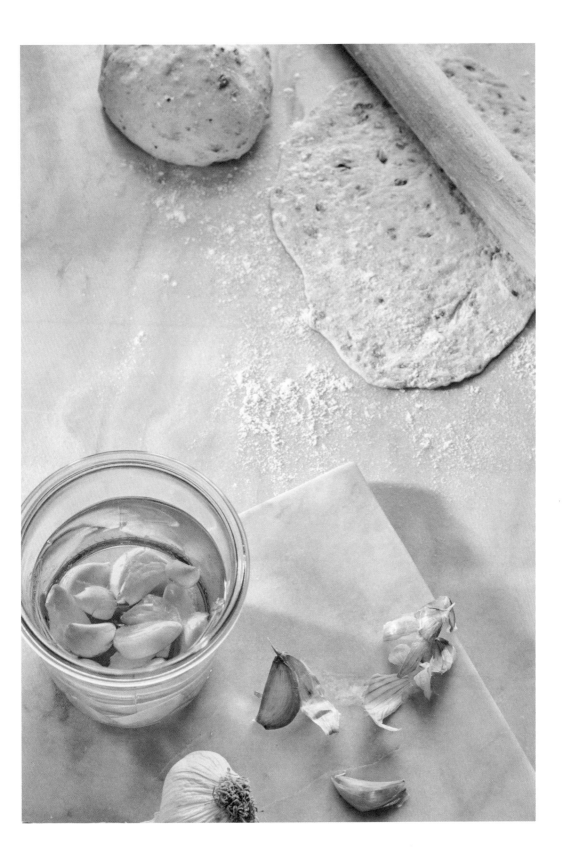

Homemade tortilla wraps

energy levels | mood regulation

HELPS WITH

Makes 8 wraps
Ready in 30 minutes

VG

250g (1⅔ cups) wholemeal
  flour, plus extra, for dusting
2 tsp olive oil
1 tsp fine sea salt
150ml (generous ½ cup)
  warm water

I have made these so many times and I'm still amazed by how easy and delicious they are. Shop-bought wholegrain or seed tortillas are decent enough options to include in your diet, but nothing beats a homemade version. Using a wholemeal flour will boost your fibre and B-vitamin intake. B vitamins are important in supporting good energy levels.

1 Put the flour, oil and salt into a bowl, pour in the water and bring together into a dough. Turn out onto a lightly floured surface and knead until smooth. Shape into a ball and leave to rest for 15–20 minutes.

2 Divide into eight pieces and roll out into thin circles. Heat a large heavy-based frying pan over a medium heat and fry in batches for 1–2 minutes each side until cooked and lightly golden.

Chicken bone broth

Makes about 1.8 litres (61fl oz)
Ready in 3 hours

GF

Chicken broths are touted as being gut-healing. While scientific validation of these claims is mixed, a homemade chicken broth is soothing and feels nourishing. It takes a while to make, but you can make it in advance and freeze for when you need it.

Bones of a roast chicken,
* broken into bits*
2.5 litres (10 cups) cold water
1 tbsp apple cider vinegar
Pinch of sea salt

1 Put all the ingredients into a large saucepan, bring up to the boil, then reduce to a bare simmer and cook gently for 2½ hours.

2 Strain through a fine sieve and allow to cool before using or freezing.

good for your soul!

HELPS WITH

Tips

Save the bones from your roasts and freeze them so you can make broth when you have time. Freeze the broth in 250-500ml (9–17fl oz) containers for up to 3 months.

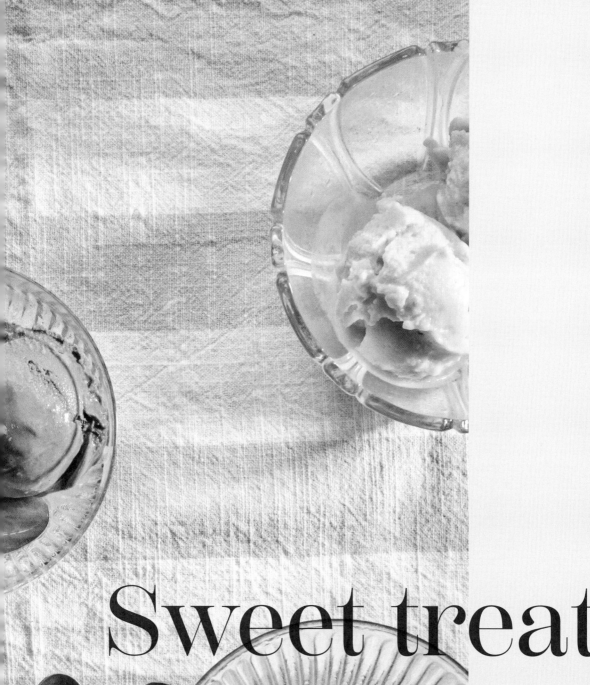

Sweet treats

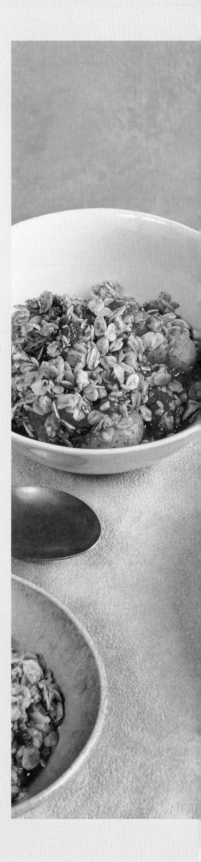

I have lived in Italy for more than five years and have first-hand experience of what the Mediterranean life entails. Italians pride themselves on cooking things from scratch. In the UK, USA and Australia, particularly when we snack, we tend to rely on ultra-processed foods like biscuits, cookies, crisps and even things that are marketed as healthier, like cereal bars. More and more research is showing us that these foods are not good for our health, particularly during the menopause when we are in extra need of nourishment. In this chapter, I share my favourite recipes that are easy to make and allow you to have a sweet delight. A little of what you fancy does you good, after all!

Chocolate-chip cookies with a secret ingredient

Makes 8–10 cookies
Ready in 30 minutes

VG GF

Chocolate-chip cookies that are good for you! A great snack option or, if you're partial to a sweet breakfast (like the Italians), this could also work. The addition of the chickpeas adds fibre and protein, which means this cookie won't spike your blood-sugar levels the way a typical cookie would.

1 x 400g (14oz) tin chickpeas, drained and rinsed
100g (scant ½ cup) peanut butter
2 tbsp ground flaxseed
2 tbsp maple syrup
1 tsp vanilla extract
100g (⅔ cup) dark (at least 70%) chocolate chips
¾ tsp baking powder

1 Preheat the oven to 180°C (350°F).

2 In a small food processor, blitz the chickpeas and peanut butter until smooth, then scoop into a bowl. Add the flaxseed, maple syrup, vanilla extract, chocolate chips and baking powder and mix well.

3 Use a small ice-cream scoop to dollop spoonfuls of the mixture onto a lined baking sheet. Press down lightly, then bake for 15 minutes until golden.

4 Allow to cool on the tray for 10 minutes, then transfer to a wire rack to cool completely.

Tips

You can use any nut butter. For extra protein, try black chickpeas. These cookies will keep in an airtight container for 2–3 days.

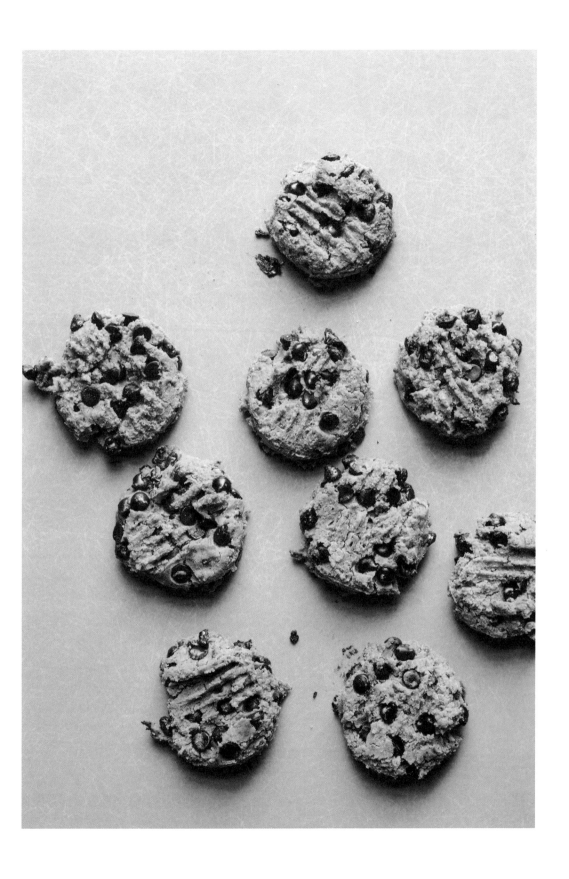

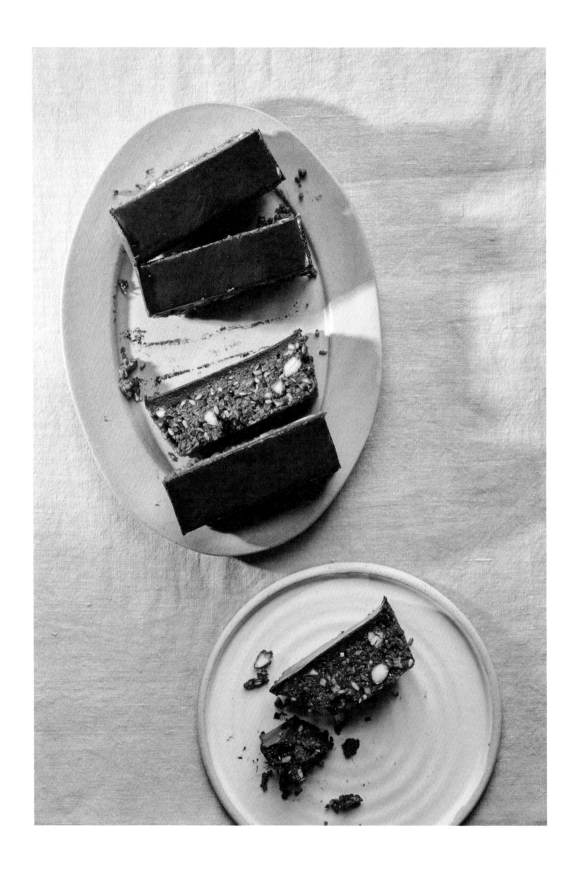

Dark chocolate crunch bars (aka 'healthy' protein bars)

Makes 10-12 bars
Ready in 20 minutes,
plus chilling

VG GF

Clients (especially those who are on the go a lot) are always asking me to recommend a protein bar. To be honest, there isn't one that I would recommend for regular consumption! They're okay as an occasional get-out-of-jail card, but not for eating more frequently. Many shop-bought protein bars hit your protein numbers, but they come with so many sweeteners and additives that aren't great for you to be eating habitually. With this recipe, I tried to create a healthy protein bar (without using protein powder) that I would be happy to recommend my clients eat regularly. Each bar gives you about 5 grams of protein – perfect for a snack. They are high in healthy fats, so, as yummy as they taste, keep it to one per snack!

2 tbsp tahini
4 tbsp almond or
  peanut butter
60g (scant ½ cup) dark (at
  least 70%) chocolate chips
200g (7oz) cooked quinoa
70g (½ cup) unpeeled
  almonds, chopped
30g (1oz) whole linseeds
  or flaxseeds

1 Line a small loaf tin or cake tin with parchment paper.

2 Either in the microwave or in a bowl set over a pan of gently simmering water, melt the tahini, nut butter and chocolate together until smooth.

3 Add the rest of the ingredients and mix well.

4 Tip into the prepared tin and chill for at least 1 hour, then cut into 10–12 small bars.

Tips

These will keep in the fridge for up to 10 days. If you like, you can drizzle with extra melted chocolate before slicing.

Chocolate and raspberry olive oil brownies

Makes 20–25 brownies
Ready in 1 hour

V GF DF

Ask me to bring something sweet to a dinner party or barbecue? I will bring these. They are my signature dish. They are simple to make and are always devoured in minutes. Nigella Lawson's olive oil chocolate cake was the inspiration, but of course I have adapted these to be as low in sugar as possible and have added more fibre. I love the visual effect of the raspberries on top.

50g (½ cup) cocoa powder
125ml (½ cup) boiling water
1 tsp vanilla bean paste
150g (1½ cups) ground almonds
½ tsp bicarbonate of soda (baking soda)
100g (scant ½ cup) caster (superfine) sugar
150ml (generous ½ cup) olive oil, plus extra, for greasing
3 large eggs
100g (generous ¾ cup) raspberries

1 Preheat the oven to 180°C (350°F). Grease a 20cm (8-inch) square brownie tin and line with parchment paper.

2 In a heatproof bowl, whisk the cocoa powder with the boiling water and vanilla.

3 In a separate bowl, mix the ground almonds with the bicarbonate of soda.

4 In a stand mixer or with a handheld electric whisk, beat the caster sugar, oil and eggs together until they are gorgeous, pale and voluminous.

5 Fold in the ground almond and cocoa mixtures, then pour into the prepared tin. Scatter over the raspberries.

6 Bake for 35–40 minutes until a skewer comes out not quite clean but not really sticky, then allow to cool in the tin before slicing into squares.

Tips

Swap the raspberries for pecans or walnuts.
These brownies will keep in an airtight container for 1–2 days.

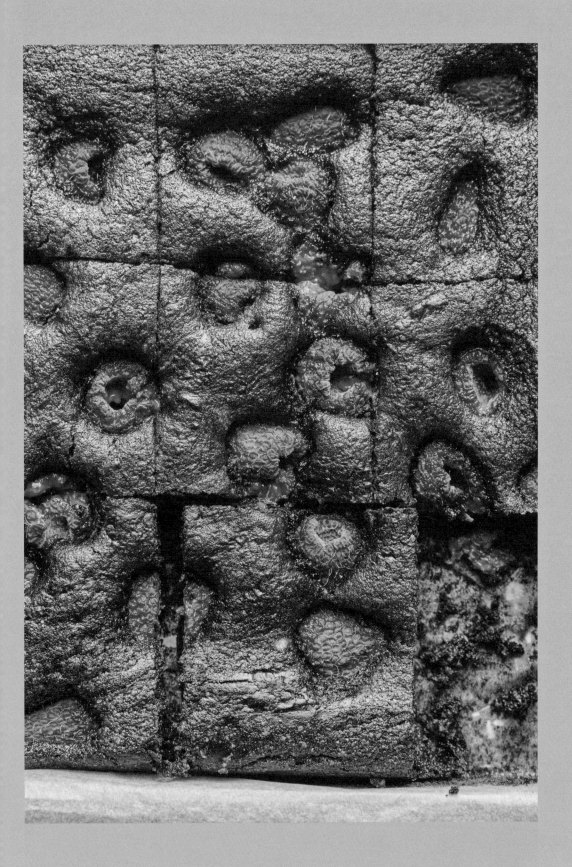

Strawberry crumble cobbler

Serves 4
Ready in 1 hour

V GF DFO

Crumbles are timeless. They can be made with all sorts of different fruits depending on what's in season. I also love that the crumble on top can be hormone-friendly. I have added some oats to boost the fibre content and flaxseeds to add some plant-based phytoestrogens, which gently top up your levels of oestrogen. The pistachios add healthy fat.

300g (10½oz) strawberries, halved
100g (scant 1 cup) raspberries
Juice of ½ orange
2 tsp cornflour (cornstarch)
2 tbsp honey
120g (1¼ cups) gluten-free jumbo rolled oats
2 tbsp soft light brown sugar
2 tbsp whole flaxseeds
50g (⅓ cup) pistachios, chopped
½ tsp ground cinnamon
Pinch of sea salt
75ml (⅓ cup) olive oil
Greek yoghurt, to serve (optional)

1 Preheat the oven to 190°C (375°F).

2 Toss the fruit with the orange juice, cornflour and honey in an ovenproof dish.

3 In a bowl, mix the oats with the sugar, flaxseeds, pistachios and cinnamon. Add a pinch of salt, then stir in the olive oil.

4 Spoon the oat mixture over the fruit and bake for 40–45 minutes until golden and brown. Serve with the yoghurt.

Tips

This crumble topping is great for any fruit. Try a classic apple crumble, adding some ground ginger to the topping, or try it with rhubarb. You can use almonds or hazelnuts instead of pistachios, or you could try it with pine nuts or pumpkin seeds (pepitas).

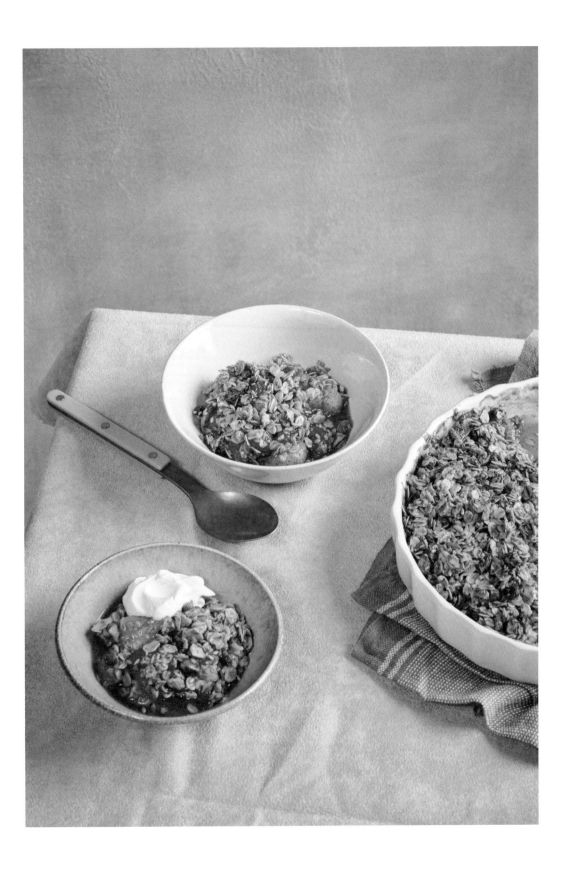

Frozen yoghurt 2 ways

If you're looking for a delicious and nutritious alternative to ice cream and sorbets, then look no further. These recipes are lower in sugar and I have packed in some plant goodness that will nourish your gut too! These icy sweet treats may also help cool you down if you're suffering from hot flushes.

Dark chocolate

Makes 300g (10½oz) yoghurt
Ready in 10 minutes, plus churning and freezing

V GF

380g (1½ cups) natural yoghurt or kefir yoghurt
4 tbsp maple syrup
2 tbsp cocoa powder
1 tsp vanilla extract
125ml (½ cup) oat milk

1 Blend all the ingredients together, tip into the bowl of an ice-cream maker and churn. Scoop into a tub and freeze.

Tips

Make this vegan by using a plant-based yoghurt. If you don't have an ice-cream maker, once the ingredients are blended, freeze in a container for 2 hours, then whisk with a handheld electric whisk and pop back into the freezer. Repeat twice more, then freeze completely.

Mango

Makes 600g (1lb 5oz) yoghurt
Ready in 10 minutes, plus freezing

V GF

2 large mangoes, chopped
1 large banana, chopped
400g (1½ cups) natural yoghurt
½ tsp ground cardamom
2 tbsp honey

Mangoes and bananas contain plenty of fibre, as well as micronutrients like vitamins A and B6.

1 Freeze the mango and banana for at least 5 hours or overnight until solid. Tip into a food processor with the yoghurt, cardamom and honey and blitz. Spoon into a tub and freeze completely.

Tip

You can also freeze the yoghurt in lollipop moulds.

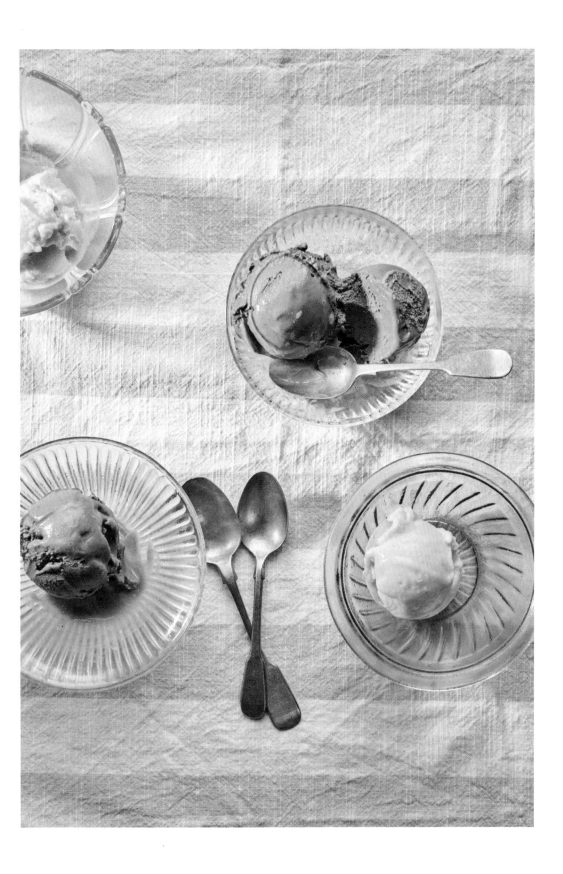

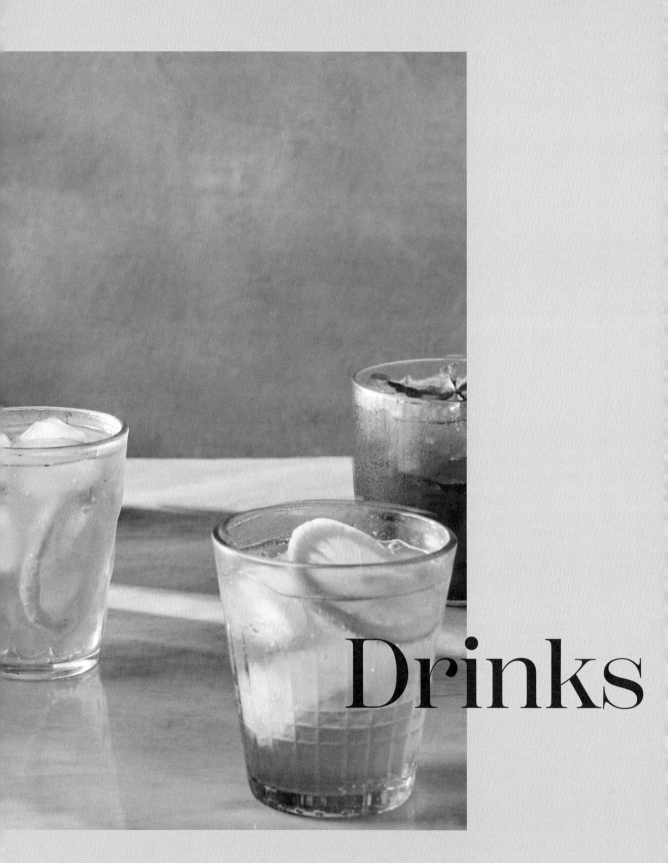

Drinks

I really wanted to add a drinks section to this book. Spoiler alert – there's no alcohol involved. The reality is that alcohol and the menopause are not the best of friends. Alcohol can worsen menopausal symptoms, from hot flushes to mood swings, and it can also make weight loss and sleep harder. However, I know that socialising is part of life, and many clients ask me for alternatives – holding a glass of sparkling water just doesn't cut it. This section of the book gives you some alcohol-free options. Please note that while there is no alcohol in these drinks, some do contain added sugar, so they should be part of your 20-per-cent indulgences.

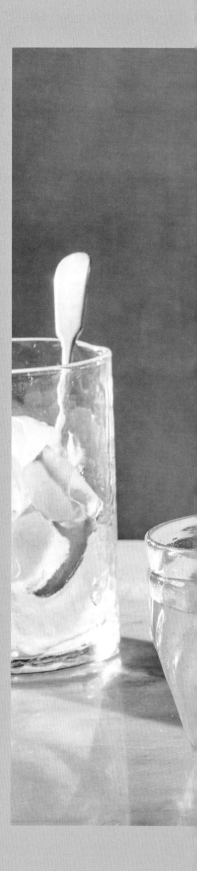

Rock shandy

Serves 2
Ready in 5 minutes

VG GF

250ml (9fl oz) soda water
200ml (7fl oz) lemonade
Few dashes of Angostura
   bitters
6 thin slices of lemon

I love bitter flavours, so I adore a rock shandy. It's so refreshing! There are an increasing number of zero-alcohol beers out there, so you can use one instead of the soda water and bitters.

1 Whisk together the soda water and lemonade.

2 Pour over ice in two glasses, adding a dash or two of bitters.

3 Garnish with lemon and serve.

Pineapple iced tea

Makes 1.75 litres (59fl oz)
Ready in 1 hour

VGO GF

1 large pineapple
1 small thumb-sized piece of
   fresh turmeric, peeled and
   sliced
3cm (1¼ inch) piece of fresh
   ginger, bashed with a rolling
   pin or pestle
Zest and juice of 1 lemon
Zest and juice of 2 oranges
1 sprig of fresh rosemary
   (optional)
1 star anise
1.75 litres (59fl oz) water
2 tbsp honey or maple syrup

Liquid gold! I was born and bred in a remote area of Zambia that is famous for its amazing pineapples. My grandmother Sara was into her natural medicine and was always cooking up herbal concoctions when we were sick. She used to tell me this one was to help my tummy feel better. I absolutely love it. It's so refreshing and feels so nourishing. Granny Sara was onto something!

1 Wash and peel the pineapple and put the flesh into a saucepan with the turmeric and ginger. Add the lemon and orange zest along with the rosemary and star anise.

2 Pour over the water, bring to the boil and simmer for 30 minutes. Allow to cool completely, then strain through a sieve, pressing to get the flavour from the pineapple.

3 Whisk in the lemon and orange juice and the honey.

Tip

This recipe leaves all the pineapple flesh for you to enjoy!

Watermelon and lime virgin mojito

Serves 4
Ready in 15 minutes

VG GF

500g (1lb 2oz) ripe
   watermelon flesh
Juice of 3 limes
100g (3½oz) bunch of fresh
   mint, leaves picked, plus
   4 sprigs, extra, to garnish
400ml (14fl oz) ginger ale
Soda water, to top up

Who doesn't love a mojito? I love the colours of this one. It's so refreshing and, ladies, we even managed to get some health-promoting phytochemicals (specifically lycopenes) into it! I love this recipe – it's soooo good! Cheers!

1 Blitz the watermelon flesh in a blender with the lime juice.

2 Muddle the mint leaves with some crushed ice in the bottom of four glasses, then pour the lime and watermelon purée over the top.

3 Top up with the ginger ale and soda water and garnish each glass with a sprig of mint.

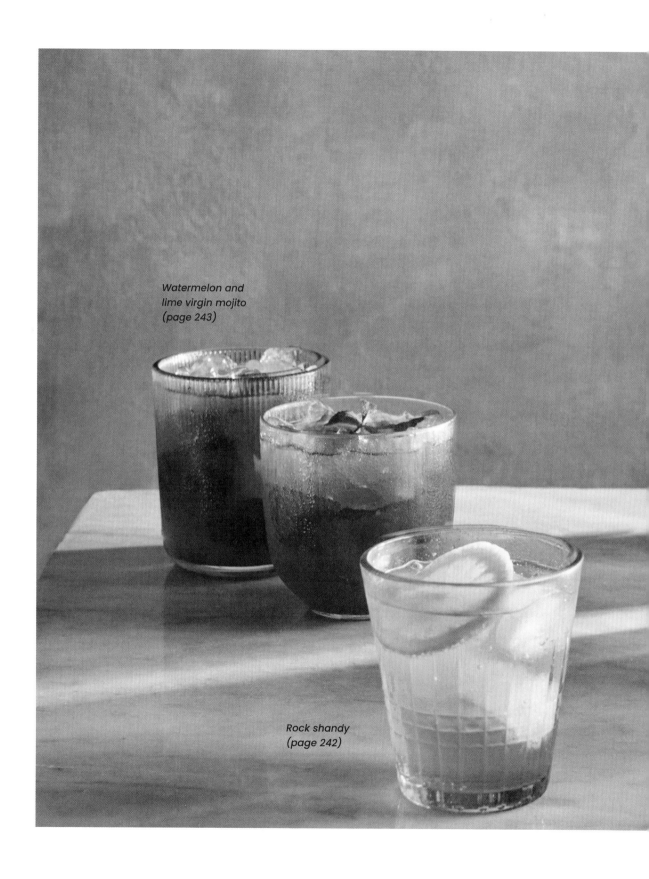

Watermelon and
lime virgin mojito
(page 243)

Rock shandy
(page 242)

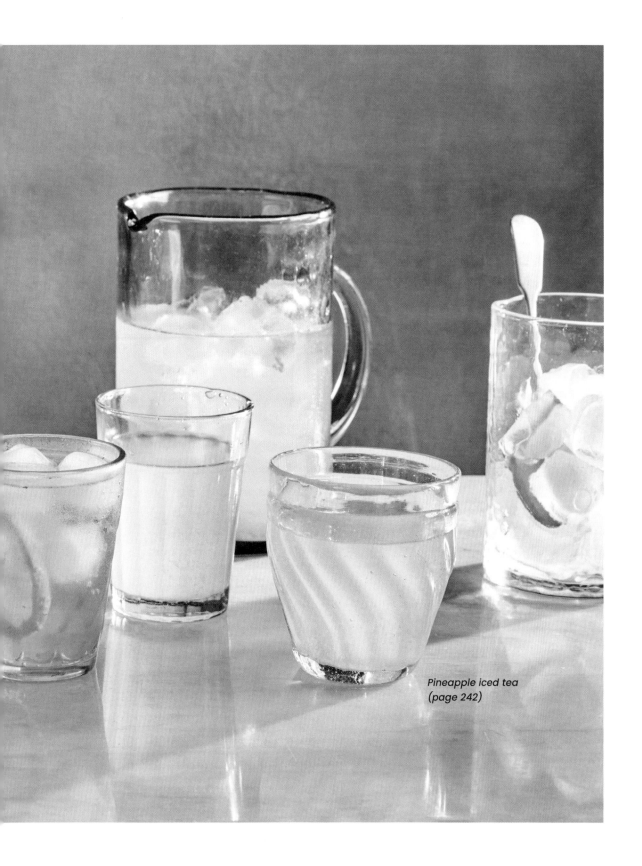

Pineapple iced tea
(page 242)

Cinnamon hot chocolate

Serves 1
Ready in 10 minutes

VG   GF

The week before my cycle, I always crave a hot chocolate. I just want the comfort. Hot chocolates are typically laden with sugar, which makes them not so good for you. I have sweetened this one naturally with dates and added cinnamon for some extra plant goodness.

300ml (10¾fl oz) milk or plant milk of choice
1 cinnamon stick or a pinch of ground cinnamon
1 large date, chopped
1½ tsp cocoa powder

1 Put the milk, cinnamon stick or powder and date into a pan over a medium heat until steaming.

2 Add the cocoa powder, remove the cinnamon stick, if using, and blend with a stick blender before serving.

Tip

Collagen powders could also work well in here. But if you're vegetarian or vegan, just remember most are based on animal sources.

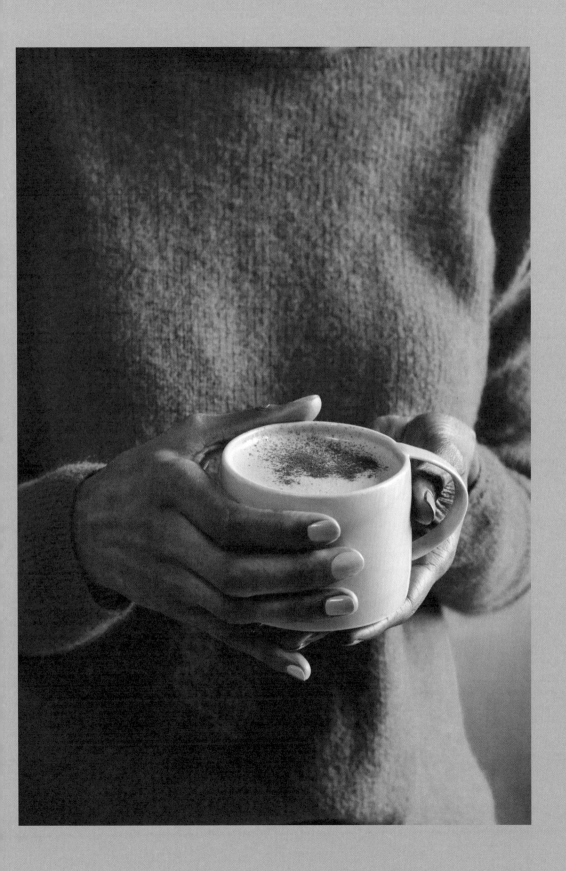

Green tea lemonade

Serves 4
Ready in 10 minutes, plus infusing

V GF DF

400ml (14fl oz) boiling water
1 green tea bag
Pared zest and juice of 1 large
    lemon
2 tbsp honey
750ml (26fl oz) sparkling
    water

I am a massive fan of green tea. It's one of my daily drinks and is bursting with antioxidants that are thought to have anti-inflammatory properties. It also has an amino acid called L-theanine, which gives you the effect of caffeine without the jitters. Pour me some more green tea, please!

1 Pour the boiling water over the green tea bag and lemon zest and allow to steep for 10 minutes, then cool completely.

2 Squeeze the lemon juice into the green tea mixture and add the honey.

3 Pour over ice into four glasses and top up with sparkling water.

Tip

Look out for green tea bags that produce a clear green tea for the best flavour and look.

Fiery ginger and chilli switchel

Makes 500ml (17fl oz)
Ready in 48 hours

V GF DF

My biggest vice is fizzy drinks. I love them! As a kid, during the school holidays, I would have a Coca-Cola or a Fanta a day, if not two, so I have an emotional association with fizzy drinks and relaxation! Luckily, adult dietitian Linia is a little wiser and knows that for optimal hormone health, sugary fizzy drinks are not great if drunk habitually – and the diet alternatives aren't that great for my gut bugs either. So, here is my labour of love! It still contains sugar (the honey) but is sooo much better for me, my gut microbiome and my hormones. A great alternative to a fizzy drink, as part of my twenty per cent.

1 whole hand of fresh ginger, peeled
300ml (10¾fl oz) boiling water
200ml (7fl oz) raw apple cider vinegar with the 'mother'
120g (⅓ cup) honey
1 small red chilli, halved lengthways
Juice of 1 lemon
Soda water or tonic water, to top up

1 Bash the ginger with a rolling pin and put it into a large jug. Pour over the boiling water and let it cool completely.

2 Add the vinegar, honey and chilli, then pour into a jar. Cover and leave to stand for 24–48 hours, then add the lemon juice and strain into a clean bottle.

3 Pour a measure (30ml/1fl oz) into a glass with ice, top up with soda water or tonic and serve.

Tips

Other flavours to try are rosemary and orange or turmeric and lemon. This keeps for 1 week in the fridge.

Appendix: Symptom checker

Go through this list and indicate the extent to which you are currently experiencing and bothered by any of these symptoms by placing a tick in the appropriate box and adding a note.

SYMPTOM	YES	NO	DETAILS
Changes to period			
Anxiety			
Feeling depressed			
Feeling tense or nervous			
Poor concentration			
Poor memory			
Brain fog			
Headaches			
Loss of confidence			
Heart palpitations			
Hot flushes			
Night sweats			
Low energy/ fatigue			
Painful joints			
Bloating			
Weight gain			
Vaginal dryness/ itching			

Notes

Introduction

1. **Page 9:** 'Another 75 per cent report not knowing...' The Fawcett Society, 2022, Menopause and the Workplace <www.fawcettsociety.org.uk/Handlers/Download.ashx?IDMF=9672cf45-5f13-4b69-8882-1e5e643ac8a6>

Chapter 1

2. **Page 13:** 'There are 200 different hormones in the human body...' Gardner, D.G., Shoback, D., 'Preface', in *Greenspan's Basic & Clinical Endocrinology*, New York NY: McGraw-Hill Education, 2017

3. **Page 17:** 'According to the American Society for Reproductive Medicine's...' Harlow, S.D., Gass, M., Hall, J.E. et al., 'Executive summary of the Stages of Reproductive Aging Workshop + 10: addressing the unfinished agenda of staging reproductive aging', The *Journal of Clinical Endocrinology and Metabolism*, 2012, vol. 97 no. 4, pp. 1159–1168

4. **Page 20:** 'Add to this the fact that science has shown...' Vassy, J.L., Meigs, J.B. 'Is genetic testing useful to predict type 2 diabetes?', *Best Practice & Research Clinical Endocrinology & Metabolism*, 2012, vol. 26 no. 2, pp. 189–201

5. **Page 20:** 'In the Western world, research shows...' Sapre, S., Thakur, R., 'Lifestyle and dietary factors determine age at natural menopause', *Journal of Mid-life Health*, 2014, vol. 5 no. 1, pp. 3–5

6. **Page 20:** 'They have also been reported to be more likely to have...' Harlow, S.D., Burnett-Bowie, S.M., Greendale, G.A. et al., 'Disparities in Reproductive Aging and Midlife Health between Black and White Women: The Study of Women's Health Across the Nation (SWAN)', *Women's Midlife Health*, 2022, vol. 8 no. 3

7. **Page 20:** 'Stressful life events, IVF treatment...' Daan, N.M., Fauser, B.C., 'Menopause prediction and potential implications', *Maturitas*, 2015, vol. 82 no. 3, pp. 257–265

8. **Page 20:** 'Stressful life events, IVF treatment...' Tao, X., Jiang, A., Yin, L. et al., 'Body mass index and age at natural menopause: a meta-analysis', *Menopause*, 2015, vol. 22 no. 4, pp. 469–474

9. **Page 20:** 'Similarly, going through IVF cycles...' Mishra, G.D., Chung, H.F., Cano, A. et al., 'EMAS position statement: Predictors of premature and early natural menopause', *Maturitas*, 2019, vol. 123, pp. 82–88

10. **Page 20:** 'Smokers reach menopause an average of...' Schoenaker, D.A., Jackson, C.A., Rowlands, J.V. et al., 'Socioeconomic position, lifestyle factors and age at natural menopause: a systematic review and meta-analyses of studies across six continents', *International Journal of Epidemiology*, 2014, vol. 43 no. 5, pp. 1542–1562

11. **Page 20:** 'However, this also means they...' Tao et al, 'Body mass index and age at natural menopause'

12. **Page 21:** 'A recent large study in the UK found...' Dunneram, Y., Greenwood, D.C., Burley, V.J. et al., 'Dietary intake and age at natural menopause: results from the UK Women's Cohort Study', *Journal of Epidemiology and Community Health*, 2018, vol. 72, pp. 733–740

13. **Page 21:** 'Research shows that the menopause transition...' Paramsothy, P., Harlow, S.D., Nan, B. et al., 'Duration of the menopausal transition is longer in women with young age at onset: the multiethnic Study of Women's Health Across the Nation', *Menopause*, 2017, vol. 24 no. 2, pp. 142–149

14. **Page 28:** 'The statistics say that on average...' Obesity Action Coalition, 2014, *The Truth about Menopause and Weight Gain* <obesityaction.org/resources/the-truth-about-menopause-and-weight-gain>

15. **Page 30:** 'Hot flushes are the classic menopause symptom...' Bansal, R., Aggarwal, N., 'Menopausal hot flashes: a concise review', *Journal of Mid-life Health*, 2019, vol. 10 no. 1, pp. 6–13

16. **Page 30:** 'Vaginal issues affect 80 per cent of women...' Simon, J.A., Kokot-Kierepa, M., Goldstein, J. et al., 'Vaginal health in the United States: results from the Vaginal Health: Insights, Views & Attitudes survey', *Menopause*, 2013, vol. 20 no. 10, pp. 1043–1048

17. **Page 32:** 'Heart disease is the number one killer of women.' Centers for Disease Control and Prevention, 2024, *Lower Your Risk for the Number 1 Killer of Women* <cdc.gov/ healthequity/features/heartdisease/index. html>

18. **Page 32:** 'Heart disease is the number one killer of women.' British Heart Foundation, 2024, *UK Factsheet* <bhf.org. uk/-/media/files/for-professionals/ research/heart-statistics/bhf-cvd- statistics-uk-factsheet.pdf>

19. **Page 32:** 'Around 10 per cent of a woman's bone mass is lost...' Nash, Z., Al-Wattar, B.H., Davies, M., 'Bone and heart health in menopause', *Best Practice & Research Clinical Obstetrics & Gynaecology*, 2022, vol. 81, pp. 61–68

20. **Page 32:** 'Alzheimer's disease is the most common type of dementia...' Dementia UK, 2022, *Alzheimer's disease* <dementiauk.org/ information-and-support/types-of- dementia/alzheimers-disease>

21. **Page 32:** 'Studies indicate that women who went through menopause prematurely...' Caldwell, J.Z.K., Isenberg, N., 'The aging brain: risk factors and interventions for long term brain health in women,' *Current Opinion in Obstetrics and Gynecology*, 2023, vol. 35 no. 2, pp. 169–175

22. **Page 32:** 'Research in rats shows that a reduction in oestrogen...' Li, R., Cui, J., Shen, Y., 'Brain sex matters: estrogen in cognition and Alzheimer's disease,' *Molecular and Cellular Endocrinology*, 2014, vol. 389 no. 1–2, pp. 13–21

Chapter 2

23. **Page 39:** 'Your entire body is 75 per cent water...' Riebl, S.K., Davy, B.M., 'The Hydration Equation: update on water balance and cognitive performance', *American College of Sports Medicine's Health & Fitness Journal*, 2013, vol. 17 no. 6, pp. 21–28

24. **Page 39:** 'Mild dehydration occurs when you experience...' Riebl et al., 'The Hydration Equation'

25. **Page 39:** 'New research using MRIs suggests...' Liu, Y., Paajanen, T., Zhang, Y. et al., 'Analysis of regional MRI volumes and thicknesses as predictors of conversion from mild cognitive impairment to Alzheimer's disease', *Neurobiology of Aging*, 2010, vol. 31 no. 8, pp. 1375–1385

26. **Page 39:** 'In a recent study, dieters who drank...' Stookey, J.D., Constant, F., Popkin, B.M. et al., 'Drinking water is associated with weight loss in overweight dieting women independent of diet and activity', *Obesity*, 2008, vol. 16 no. 11, pp. 2481–2488

27. **Page 40:** 'As a guide, you should drink...' The Association of UK Dietitians, 2023, *Fluid (water and drinks) and hydration* <bda. uk.com/resource/fluid-water-drinks.html>

28. **Page 42:** 'Caffeine is a stimulant...' van Dam, R.M., Hu, F.B., Willett, W.C., 'Coffee, Caffeine, and Health', *The New England Journal of Medicine*, 2020, vol. 383 no. 4, pp. 369–378

29. **Page 42:** 'A recent study of 2507 menopausal women...' Faubion, S.S., Sood, R., Thielen, J.M. et al., 'Caffeine and menopausal symptoms: what is the association?', *Menopause*, 2015, vol. 22 no. 2, pp. 155–158

30. **Page 42:** 'Daily caffeine limits...' European Food Safety Authority, 2015, *Caffeine* <efsa. europa.eu/en/topics/topic/caffeine>

31. **Page 44:** 'Current UK guidelines recommend...' The Association of UK Dietitians, 2023, *Nutrients food facts* <bda.uk.com/food-health/food-facts/ nutrients-food-facts.html>

32. **Page 50:** 'The current guidelines are to reduce your sugar intake...' The Association of UK Dietitians, 2023, *Nutrients food facts* <bda.uk.com/food-health/food-facts/nutrients-food-facts.html>

33. **Page 53:** 'A 2021 study that compared women...' Ko, J., Park, Y.M., 'Menopause and the loss of skeletal muscle mass in women', *Iranian Journal of Public Health*, 2021, vol. 50 no. 2, pp. 413–414

34. **Page 53:** 'Physiologically, bones are not just...' Clarke, B., 'Normal bone anatomy and physiology', *Clinical Journal of the American Society of Nephrology*, 2008, no. 3, pp. 131–139

35. **Page 54:** 'Recommendations are that we have...' World Cancer Research Fund International, *Limit Red and Processed Meat* <wcrf.org/diet-activity-and-cancer/cancer-prevention-recommendations/limit-red-and-processed-meat>

36. **Page 54:** 'In the UK, for adults...' The Association of UK Dietitians, 2023, *All Food Fact Pages* <bda.uk.com/food-health/food-facts/all-food-fact-sheets.html>

37. **Page 54:** 'There are no specific protein guidelines for menopausal women...' Bruyère, O., Honvo, G., Veronese, N. et al., 'An updated algorithm recommendation for the management of knee osteoarthritis from the European Society for Clinical and Economic Aspects of Osteoporosis, Osteoarthritis and Musculoskeletal Diseases (ESCEO)', *Seminars in Arthritis and Rheumatism*, 2019, vol. 49 no. 3, pp. 337–350

38. **Page 58:** 'Within this, we are advised...' British Nutrition Foundation, 2023, *Fat* <nutrition.org.uk/healthy-sustainable-diets/fat/?level=Consumer>

39. **Page 58:** 'Trans fats should be kept to a minimum...' British Nutrition Foundation, *Fat*

40. **Page 58:** 'It's recommended that we eat...' NHS, 2022, *Fish and shellfish* <www.nhs.uk/live-well/eat-well/food-types/fish-and-shellfish-nutrition>

41. **Page 58:** 'One portion is approximately...' The Association of UK Dietitians, 2023, *All Food Fact Pages* <bda.uk.com/food-health/food-facts/all-food-fact-sheets.html>

42. **Page 61:** 'During the menopause, hormonal changes...' Siddiqui, R., Makhlouf, Z., Alharbi, A.M. et al., 'The Gut Microbiome and Female Health', *Biology*, 2022, vol. 11 no. 11

43. **Page 61:** 'From my clinical experience...' Elli, L., Branchi, F., Tomba, C. et al., 'Diagnosis of gluten related disorders: Celiac disease, wheat allergy and non-celiac gluten sensitivity', *World Journal of Gastroenterology*, 2015, vol. 21 no. 23, pp. 7110–7119

44. **Page 62:** 'Roughly 95 per cent of your body's serotonin...' Gao, K., Mu, C.L., Farzi, A. et al., 'Tryptophan metabolism: a link between the gut microbiota and brain', *Advances in Nutrition*, 2020, vol. 11 no. 3, pp. 709–723

45. **Page 66:** 'American researchers found that people who ate...' McDonald, D., Hyde, E., Debelius, J.W. et al., 'American gut: an open platform for citizen science microbiome research', *mSystems*, 2018, vol. 3 no. 3, pp. 10–1128

46. **Page 74:** 'We also don't know how different population groups...' Vigar, V., Myers, S., Oliver, C. et al., 'A systematic review of organic versus conventional food consumption: is there a measurable benefit on human health?', *Nutrients*, 2019, vol. 12 no. 7

47. **Page 74:** 'We also don't know how different population groups...' Gerasimidis, K., Bryden, K., Chen, X. et al., 'The impact of food additives, artificial sweeteners and domestic hygiene products on the human gut microbiome and its fibre fermentation capacity', *European Journal of Nutrition*, 2020, vol. 59, pp. 3213–3230

48. **Page 74:** 'We also don't know how different population groups...' Neff, A.M., Laws, M.J., Warner, G.R. et al., 'The effects of environmental contaminant exposure on reproductive aging and the menopause transition', *Current Environmental Health Reports*, 2022, vol. 9, pp. 53–79

49. **Page 74:** 'We also don't know how different population groups...' Schmidt, C.W., 'Age at menopause: do chemical exposures play a role?', *Environmental Health Perspectives*, 2017, vol. 125 no. 6

50. **Page 74:** 'We also don't know how different population groups...' Grindler, N.M., Allsworth, J.E., Macones, G.A. et al., 'Persistent organic pollutants and early menopause in U.S. women', *PLoS One*, 2015, vol. 10 no. 1

51. **Page 74:** 'We also don't know how different population groups...' Vahter, M., Berglund, M., Akesson, Å., 'Toxic metals and the menopause', *British Menopause Society Journal*, 2004, vol. 10 no. 2, pp. 60–64

Chapter 3

52. **Page 84:** 'About 75 per cent of women in the Western world...' Bansal, R., 'Menopausal hot flashes'

53. **Page 85:** 'Menopause and alcohol...' Hendriks, H.F.J., 'Alcohol and human health: what is the evidence?', *Annual Review of Food Science and Technology*, 2020, vol. 11, pp. 1–21

54. **Page 85:** 'Menopause and alcohol...' He, S., Hasler, B.P., Chakravorty, S., 'Alcohol and sleep-related problems', *Current Opinion in Psychology*, 2019, vol. 30, pp. 117–122

55. **Page 85:** 'Menopause and alcohol...' Bonanni, E., Schirru, A., Di Perri, M.C. et al., 'Insomnia and hot flashes', *Maturitas*, 2019, vol. 126, 51–54

56. **Page 85:** 'It's easy to lose track of how much you are drinking...' The Association of UK Dietitians, 2023, *Nutrients food facts*

57. **Page 87:** 'It's recommended that we do at least 150 minutes...' NHS, *Exercise* <www.nhs.uk/live-well/exercise>

58. **Page 88:** 'Around 10 per cent of a woman's bone mass...' Nash, Z., 'Bone and heart health in menopause'

SCAN THIS QR CODE TO UNLOCK A COMPREHENSIVE LISTING OF SOURCE MATERIAL THAT UNDERPINS THE RESEARCH FOR THIS BOOK.

Resources

General menopause information

United Kingdom

Black Health and Beyond, blackhealthandbeyond.co.uk

The British Menopause Society, thebms.org.uk

Daisy Network (a charity for women with premature menopause), daisynetwork.org

Menopause Cafe, menopausecafe.net

The Menopause Charity, themenopausecharity.org

South Asian Women's Health Group, fareehajay.com

North America

Black Girl's Guide to Surviving Menopause, blackgirlsguidetosurvivingmenopause.com

Let's Talk Menopause, letstalkmenopause.org

The North American Menopause Society, menopause.org

Red Hot Mamas, redhotmamas.org

Australia

Australasian Menopause Society, menopause.org.au

Breathing specialists (UK)

Michael James Wong, justbreatheproject.com

Rebecca Dennis, breathingtree.co.uk

Counselling and Psychotherapy (UK)

Beat Eating Disorders, beateatingdisorders.org.uk

British Association for Counselling and Psychotherapy, bacp.co.uk

Psychiatric & Psychological Consultant Services, ppcsltd.co.uk

Nutrition experts (UK)

Bloom Health Hub, bloomhealthhub.com

British Dietetic Association, bda.uk.com/find-a-dietitian.html

Tracy Kelly, Women's Health Dietitian, tracykellysays.com

VMW Nutrition, vmwnutrition.co.uk

Medical and lifestyle management (UK)

Dr Elise Dallas, thelondongeneralpractice.com

Pure Sports Medicine, puresportsmed.com

Mindful meditation (UK and USA)

Dr Tara Swart, taraswart.com

Yoga Mama, yogamama.co.uk

Movement specialists (UK)

The Putney Clinic of Physical Therapy, putneyclinic.co.uk

Warrior Sports Rehabilitation, warriorsportsrehab.com

Pelvic floor specialists (UK)

Louise Buttler, Live Brave Pilates, livebrave.life

Powerhouse Pilates (Pascale Falempin) powerhousepilates.it

Sleep (UK and USA)

Dr Shelby Harris, drshelbyharris.com

The Sleep Foundation, sleepfoundation.org

Index

Acknowledgements

Saying thank you to all the people who have helped to bring this book to life feels like an overwhelming task. I could write another whole book! It takes a village to write a book and I am ever so grateful for mine.

A massive thank you Tess for your support and encouragement with this project. You are an absolute gem and are much appreciated.

Borra, Jan, Meghan and the amazing team at DML Talent, I am honoured to be part of the family.

The work that goes into a book is insane. What a pleasure it has been to work with the team at Murdoch Books. Céline, Virginia, Megan, Claire, Clare, Rachel, Gina and Kay, what superstars you all are. You embraced all the ideas and took them up a level and kept things moving seamlessly. I loved the energy and how excited we all got seeing the book come to life. A huge thank you also to Lizzie and Georgie for their abundance of skills in perfecting recipes and styling the food. I am so proud of what we have all created. Thank you.

I have access to the best nutritional science sounding board. Sasha, Tracy and Victoria, I was extremely demanding of your time and expertise. The many phone calls and messages at all hours of the day were invaluable. Thank you. Shout out also to my dietitian colleagues Fiona, Jo and Janey for your practical perspectives and proofing. A big appreciation to my medical colleagues Elise, Adam and Fred for your medical touches.

Last but never least: my tribe. A big thank you to my family and friends. What a blessing you all are! You love, you support, you provide a home from home, you fill in my surveys, you give ideas, you taste, you challenge, you check in and you help refill my bucket over and over. You are the reason I could write this book with such a tight deadline and stay semi-sane. A special thank you to my sisters from another mister, Nasima and Sherrie-Lyn. You are my biggest cheerleaders and my personal proofreaders. Ari, my dear friend who doubles as a sounding board and tells me as it is – your input in the tone of this project was of great value. And, of course, a shout-out to Rabih, who thinks he should be the co-author! Thank you for my mountain writing pad. You have also been instrumental in my thought process for this book. You bring creativity to my thinking and constantly encourage me to think outside the box. Thank you.

Published in 2024 by Murdoch Books,
an imprint of Allen & Unwin

Murdoch Books UK
Ormond House
26–27 Boswell Street
London WC1N 3JZ
Phone: +44 (0) 20 8785 5995
murdochbooks.co.uk
info@murdochbooks.co.uk

Murdoch Books Australia
Cammeraygal Country
83 Alexander Street
Crows Nest NSW 2065
Phone: +61 (0)2 8425 0100
murdochbooks.com.au
info@murdochbooks.com.au

For corporate orders and custom publishing,
contact our business development team at
salesenquiries@murdochbooks.com.au

Publisher: Céline Hughes
Editorial manager: Virginia Birch
Design manager: Megan Pigott
Designer: Claire Rochford
Editor: Gina Flaxman
Recipe editor: Kay Delves
Photographer: Clare Winfield
Stylist: Rachel Vere
Food editor and home economist:
  Lizzie Kamenetzky
Production director, Australia: Lou Playfair
Production director, UK: Niccolò De Bianchi

Text © Linia Patel 2024
The moral right of the author has
been asserted.
Design © Murdoch Books 2024
Photography © Clare Winfield 2024

Every reasonable effort has been made to trace the owners of
copyright materials in this book, but in some instances this has
proven impossible. The author(s) and publisher will be glad to
receive information leading to more complete acknowledgements
in subsequent printings of the book and in the meantime extend
their apologies for any omissions.

*Murdoch Books Australia acknowledges the Traditional Owners of
the Country on which we live and work. We pay our respects to all
Aboriginal and Torres Strait Islander Elders, past and present.*

All rights reserved. No part of this publication may be reproduced,
stored in a retrieval system or transmitted in any form or by any
means, electronic, mechanical, photocopying, recording or
otherwise, without the prior written permission of the publisher.

ISBN 978 1 76150 030 5

A catalogue record for this book is available from the British Library

A catalogue record for this
book is available from the
National Library of Australia

Colour reproduction by Born Group, London, UK
Printed by 1010 Printing International Limited, China

DISCLAIMER: The content presented in this book is meant for
inspiration and informational purposes only. The purchaser of
this book understands that the information contained within is
not intended to replace personalised medical advice or to be
relied upon to treat, cure or prevent any disease, illness or
medical condition. It is understood that you will seek full medical
clearance by a licensed physician before making any changes
mentioned in this book. The author and publisher claim no
responsibility to any person or entity for any liability, loss or
damage caused or alleged to be caused directly or indirectly as
a result of the use, application or interpretation of the material in
this book.

OVEN GUIDE: You may find cooking times vary depending on
the oven you are using. The recipes in this book are based on
conventional oven temperatures. For fan-assisted ovens, as
a general rule, set the oven temperature to 20°C (35°F) lower
than indicated in the recipe.

TABLESPOON MEASURES: We have used 15 ml (3 teaspoon)
tablespoon measures. If you are using a 20 ml (4 teaspoon)
tablespoon, please adjust amounts accordingly.

10 9 8 7 6 5 4 3 2 1

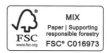